An Introduction to Infectious Diseases

Barry C. Fox, M.D.

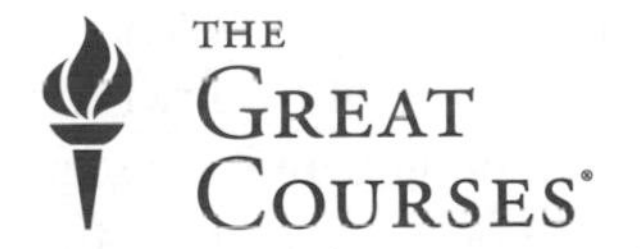

PUBLISHED BY:

THE GREAT COURSES
Corporate Headquarters
4840 Westfields Boulevard, Suite 500
Chantilly, Virginia 20151-2299
Phone: 1-800-832-2412
Fax: 703-378-3819
www.thegreatcourses.com

Printed in the United States of America

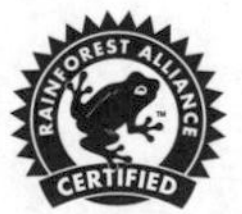

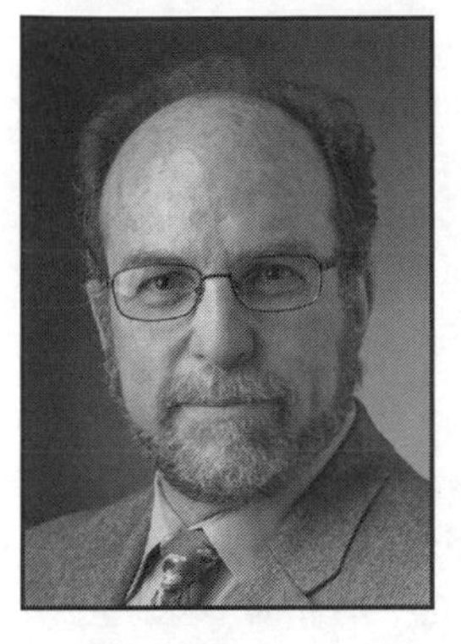

Barry C. Fox, M.D.

Clinical Professor of Infectious Disease
University of Wisconsin School of Medicine and Public Health

Dr. Barry C. Fox is a Clinical Professor of Infectious Disease at the University of Wisconsin School of Medicine and Public Health in Madison, Wisconsin. He currently practices in clinical infectious disease at two hospitals and a long-term care facility. He received his undergraduate degree in Molecular Biophysics and Biochemistry from Yale University and his medical degree from Vanderbilt University. He is board certified in both Internal Medicine and Infectious Disease.

Dr. Fox spent two years at Ohio State University as a Clinical Assistant Professor, also serving as the Head of Infection Control and Hospital Epidemiology of the Arthur G. James Cancer Hospital and Richard J. Solove Research Institute. He then spent eight years as the Head of Infectious Disease at the Carle Clinic in Urbana, Illinois, where he served as Clinical Associate Professor and in other educational capacities at the University of Illinois College of Medicine. In 2000, he returned to the University of Wisconsin.

Dr. Fox is a fellow in the Infectious Diseases Society of America and is a member of the Emerging Infectious Network. He also was elected as a fellow for the Society of Healthcare Epidemiology of America. Dr. Fox was an avid participant in the Centers for Disease Control and Prevention program known as Get Smart about Antibiotics, chairing many committees for the Wisconsin Antibiotic Resistance Network. He continues as a member of the worldwide Alliance for the Prudent Use of Antibiotics.

Dr. Fox is extensively involved in medical educational efforts, including giving lectures and organizing discussion groups on infectious diseases at the University of Wisconsin School of Medicine and Public Health, teaching advanced trainees at all levels, and giving presentations to staff at various hospitals and to organizations throughout Wisconsin. He also was the Director of Medical Education at the Internal Medicine Residency Program in Urbana, Illinois. He was named the Medical Educator of the Year by the Department of Medicine at the University of Illinois College of Medicine in 1994 and was chosen by the Internal Medicine Residency Program as the Attending of the Year in 1991.

Dr. Fox has been chosen numerous times as a Top Doc by *Madison Magazine*. On a national level, he has been recognized as one of the Best Doctors in America and made the list of America's Top Physicians compiled by the Consumer Research Council of America. In addition to patient care, he leads the Antimicrobial Stewardship Team at UW Health, the health system for University of Wisconsin Hospital and Clinics.

Dr. Fox has authored or coauthored 4 book chapters and 46 articles in a wide assortment of peer-reviewed journals; he also has presented abstracts and given presentations to international audiences on more than 30 occasions. In addition, he serves as a peer reviewer for medical journals. ■

Table of Contents

INTRODUCTION

LECTURE GUIDES

Table of Contents

Table of Contents

Acknowledgment

Special thanks to Linda Fox for course development.

Disclaimer

These lectures are not designed for use as medical references to diagnose, treat, or prevent medical illnesses or trauma, and neither The Teaching Company nor the lecturer is responsible for your use of this educational material or its consequences. Furthermore, participating in this course does not create a doctor-patient relationship. The information contained in these lectures is not intended to dictate what constitutes reasonable, appropriate, or best care for any given health issue, nor does it take into account the unique circumstances that define the health issues of the viewer. If you have questions about the diagnosis, treatment, or prevention of a medical condition or illness, you should consult your personal physician. The opinions and positions provided in these lectures reflect the opinions and positions of the relevant lecturer and do not necessarily reflect the opinions or positions of The Teaching Company or its affiliates.

The Teaching Company expressly DISCLAIMS LIABILITY for any DIRECT, INDIRECT, INCIDENTAL, SPECIAL, OR CONSEQUENTIAL DAMAGES OR LOST PROFITS that result directly or indirectly from the use of these lectures. In states that do not allow some or all of the above limitations of liability, liability shall be limited to the greatest extent allowed by law.

An Introduction to Infectious Diseases

Scope:

This course will take you on a voyage through the fascinating world of infectious diseases. You will travel through the centuries and right up to current outbreaks of new, emerging, and often deadly diseases. You will travel side by side with germs as they hitch rides by land, sea, and air, spreading their virulence worldwide. With many germs around us daily, this course will identify the beneficial ones and help you avoid or destroy the ones that cause disease.

The course begins with a scientific foundation—how bacteria, viruses, fungi, and hybrid germs invade our bodies, how they transmit disease, and what treatment can be used to fight them. You will discover how the inner components of pathogens work together to cause disease or to evade our immune systems. The means at our disposal to stop these invaders are changing rapidly, and you will learn how and why we may be losing the battle against some germs. You will study how rapid germ mutations are challenging our disease diagnosis and treatments and how this leads to antibiotic resistance. You also will examine the development of vaccines and their important role in the prevention of serious diseases, as well as their effect on global health.

Next, you will discover that wildlife—such as birds, bats, and deer—are often the source of infectious diseases. You will explore vectors of disease transmission, such as fleas, ticks, and mosquitoes. You will delve into how our interactions with wildlife and the environment affect our health, and you will learn how doctors, veterinarians, and environmentalists are working together on the One Health Initiative as a collaborative approach to improve the health of all species. You will examine exotic new diseases that are emerging from sources that were not previously thought to transmit diseases to humans.

Our organ systems are vital to our survival, and they are vulnerable to assaults by many different germs. You will examine the various infectious diseases that can affect our brains, respiratory and circulatory systems, skin, and intestinal and urinary tracts. You will get a behind-the-scenes look inside a hospital and discover the special germs lurking there—you will even be advised to try to stay out of the hospital to avoid them!

Then, you will examine some of the top infectious disease killers in the world, including human immunodeficiency virus (HIV), tuberculosis, and malaria. You also will discover why these diseases are still killing thousands daily in our era of modern medicine.

Also concerning is the potential to use pathogens as weapons for a bioterrorist attack—perhaps with diseases that are eradicated but stored in lab facilities in various countries. You will learn about historical attacks and the agents that are most concerning for future attacks.

New technologies are quickly changing the face of global disease surveillance, and you will be introduced to specialized systems and new technologies that work around the clock to keep us all safe. You will learn how social media is becoming more important for surveillance. You also will discover some great preventive information about traveling, as well as some tools to keep you healthy during your trip.

Next, you will study some of the worst public health disasters in history, such as the 1918 influenza pandemic, and examine ways to prevent or contain future health disasters. You also will go on a journey around the world, looking at clusters of disease that turn into epidemics or even worldwide pandemics. Finally, you will try to figure out what the next disease pandemic will be.

This course gives you a comprehensive historical and current perspective on infectious diseases. You will learn about the perpetual challenges we face together in the future as new diseases emerge and evolve and as old infectious diseases reemerge. By the end of this course, you will have a solid foundation of scientific knowledge about disease-causing germs—as well as disease transmission, treatments, and prevention—and the serious issues we face at home and abroad. ■

The Dynamic World of Infectious Disease

Lecture 1

The spread of infectious diseases, both past and present, is largely dependent on our interaction with one another, the environments we live in, and even our interactions with the animal world. In this lecture, you will learn about three diseases—plague and malaria, which are two of the oldest infectious diseases, and polio, a disease of the mid-1900s—that greatly impacted the state of public health, often spreading throughout countries and continents unchecked. Many people suffered and died due to the lack of knowledge about germ theory, or the lack of tools to diagnose illnesses.

Plague

- Infectious diseases have played a significant role in changing the course of human history. The Black Death, also known as the plague, originated in the Yunnan province in southwest China in 200 B.C. and was spread by Italian merchant ships to the rest of Europe in the 1300s. It swept through Europe, the Middle East, and Africa and was one of the greatest health disasters in recorded history. Estimates are that nearly 200 million people worldwide died of the plague and that it took Europe four centuries for its population to recover.

- In one form of plague, known as bubonic plague, the victim's lymph nodes became hugely swollen and were called buboes, giving the bubonic plague its name. Buboes were hard, painful, burning lumps. They often turned black—hence spawning the name the Black Plague—split open, and oozed pus. This disease was incredibly painful, and patients rarely survived more than three to four days before dying. Antibiotics were not discovered until the 1940s, so death was imminent.

- In the 1900s, the plague even spread to the United States via rats aboard steamships that had sailed from infected areas. This resulted in about 1,000 cases in the United States, primarily in the western states, and where sporadic cases still occur today. But most present-day cases of the plague occur in rural Africa—a few thousand yearly.

- Where did the plague come from, and how did it spread? Theories abounded, including the Miasma theory that bad air, poor hygiene, and contaminated water were the cause. This was the predominant theory of disease transmission until the 1860s. Some interesting, but naïve, treatments for plague included witchcraft, lancing the lymph nodes, and exotic concoctions to put on the lymph nodes.

- In the 1800s, the founder of modern-day nursing, Florence Nightingale, was one of the staunchest believers that filth and unsanitary conditions were a prime component of disease transmission. She brought strict new sanitation standards into areas filled with plague and malaria.

- It became clear that the plague was contagious, but up until the mid-19th century, the concept of germ theory did not exist. Five centuries after the plague appeared, with the invention of the microscope, we were able to identify microscopic organisms—germs—as the culprits. With this discovery of microorganisms, we celebrate France's Louis Pasteur and Germany's Robert Koch for learning to assign a specific microbe as the cause of a specific disease.

- Over time, we have learned that disease outbreaks are sometimes caused by bacteria, or viruses like influenza, or parasites like malaria. We are now able, with modern technology, to determine the causes of most infectious diseases.

- During an outbreak of the plague in Hong Kong, Pasteur sent Alexandre Yersin to try to identify the germ. He drew fluid from a dead man's buboes and looked at it under the microscope. He identified a bacterium, later named after him, called *Yersinia pestis*. Next, he injected the germ into guinea pigs. The pigs died a few days later, and he became convinced that he had identified the plague germ. He also tested some of the many dead street rats and found they contained the same bacteria.

- Pasteur sent a French army physician, Paul-Louis Simond, to figure out the vector of transmission. Simond determined that the real culprit for disease transmission was a flea, which fed on a rodent that carried the bacteria. The flea became the vector of the disease, transmitting it from animals to humans.

- The plague was so difficult to eliminate because it could remain alive and potently deadly even up to three days later in a dead body. In addition, there are more than 80 species of fleas that can transmit plague. Fortunately, with the control of flea vectors, and with antibiotics given in a timely manner, today we can cure 85 percent of plague cases.

Malaria

- Malaria is a dangerous parasitic disease that has had a tremendous global impact. Malaria is a parasite transmitted by mosquito bites that affects the functioning of our red blood cells, which control oxygen delivery to the body. Malaria is one of the oldest infectious diseases—nearly half a million years old.

- We have had plenty of time, over thousands of years, to conquer malaria, yet malaria still manages to infect one out of every 21 human beings on the planet and 300 million humans yearly. It kills nearly 1 million humans year after year. While the vast majority of global malaria mortality is in Africa, malaria still frequently occurs in Southeast Asia and the Amazon region of South America.

- During the building of the Panama Canal in the early 1900s, the wet and hot environment was the perfect breeding ground for both malaria and a viral illness called yellow fever to take hold. Malaria killed more than 30,000 workers.

- In 1897, the link between mosquitoes and malaria disease transmission was proven, and Dr. William Gorgas set out to eradicate the insects by eliminating standing water, pouring oil on immature malaria forms called larvae, and fumigating living spaces.

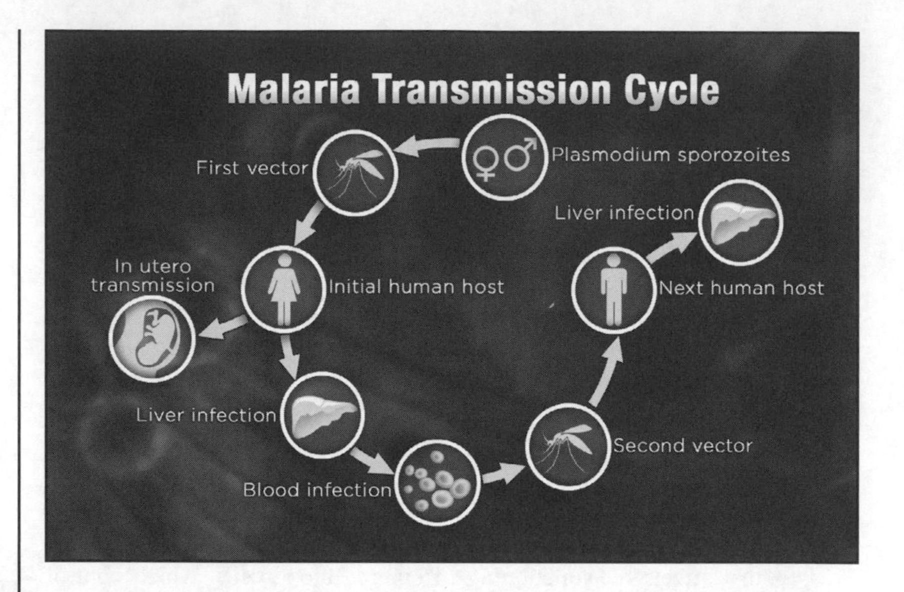

- The reason malaria is so difficult to eradicate is that there is a continuous cycle of infection occurring. First, the infected mosquitoes, carrying the malaria parasite, bite a human and inject the parasite, causing illness. Meanwhile, another mosquito that is not infected bites a human who is infected, and the mosquito becomes a new carrier, continuing the cycle of transmission.

- Environmental factors such as global warming are thought to predict a dismal future for malaria, which thrives in a warm environment. This makes for an uncertain future for malaria. There are ongoing efforts today by the World Health Organization (WHO) to try to prevent and reduce malaria illness. However, in spite of all our current efforts, one child still dies every minute from malaria in Africa.

- Unfortunately, as a harbinger of the problems with antibiotic resistance, mosquitoes have developed resistance to treatment drugs from widespread misuse. The mosquitoes also seem resilient to widespread pesticide applications, even DDT. This is a preventable and curable disease that is still causing unacceptable death rates.

Polio

- Poliomyelitis is a newer infectious disease of epidemic proportions of the 20th century. In the summer of 1916, 27,000 Americans died, 80 percent of which were children under the age of five. In 1921, Franklin Delano Roosevelt acquired polio. Seven years after contracting the illness, he founded the National Institute for Infantile Paralysis, transforming the landscape of polio research. The foundation, which later changed its name to the March of Dimes, was the first private, large-scale effort against a single disease.

- Not until the 1930s, with the invention of the electron microscope, did scientists identify this mysterious virus. It struck quickly without warning, causing mass hysteria among the people of a community that it invaded.

- Polio was first described in the medical literature several hundred years ago. Polio is actually an intestinal viral infection. It is spread from person to person through contact with fecal waste, unwashed hands, shared objects, and contaminated food and water. Poliovirus enters the body through the mouth, travels into the digestive tract, and is eventually excreted.

- Surprisingly, the most common infection the virus produces is an asymptomatic infection—meaning with no signs or symptoms, or with minor symptoms such as nausea and headache. But in a small percentage of cases, the virus travels via the bloodstream to the brain or spinal cord, destroying nerve cells called motor neurons, which are responsible for stimulating muscles to contract.

- The extent and permanence of the resulting paralysis is difficult to predict, because some infected nerve cells will fight off the virus while others will die. At its worst, polio causes irreversible paralysis, most often in the legs. The majority of deaths occurred when breathing muscles were immobilized.

- Patients were kept alive on machines known as iron lungs, an early feat of biomedical engineering that confined patients to a tank respirator. The first iron lung was developed in 1927 at Harvard University, and this invention was responsible for saving many lives during the peak of the polio epidemic.

- In addition, there was an intense effort to develop a vaccine against polio. In 1953, just after an epidemic year in which 58,000 new cases of polio were reported, an American medical researcher, Dr. Jonas Salk, announced that he had successfully tested a polio vaccine from killed virus strains.

- After conducting clinical trials on more than 2 million school children, as well as himself and his family, the vaccine was deemed safe and effective. It was widely distributed, and the total number of polio cases dropped below 6,000 in the United States in 1957, the first year the vaccine was widely available.

- In 1962, another scientist, Albert Sabin, developed a live virus weakened oral vaccine. This vaccine had to be tested abroad because Salk had his vaccine entrenched in the United States. Sabin was able to conduct an extensive polio vaccine trial in the Soviet Union at the height of the Cold War because the fear of polio was stronger than political differences. In the first five months of 1959, 10 million children in the Soviet Union received the Sabin oral vaccine, and he received a medal in gratitude from the Russian government. Both scientists donated the rights to their vaccines, unpatented, as gifts to humanity.

- In the 1960s, the Sabin oral live vaccine would supersede the Salk vaccine in the United States and, eventually, worldwide. In 1987, the WHO launched a global initiative to eradicate polio from the planet within 15 years.

- Because remaining worldwide cases were in limited geographic areas of Asia and Africa, there was reason for optimism. By the year 2000, there were fewer than 2,000 cases worldwide. As of 2012, as a result of the global effort to eradicate the disease, only three countries—Afghanistan, Nigeria, and Pakistan—had polio cases. This was reduced from more than 125 countries in 1988.

- Paradoxically, during the course of live vaccinations, there were actual cases of polio that were caused by the poliovirus live vaccine. Therefore, in the United States, the vaccine was reverted to an efficient killed version of the vaccine like the Salk vaccine. However, even in 2013, eradication of polio remained elusive, and the virus was spreading via international travel. In spite of knowing the epidemiology of the disease, the world's population is still at risk.

- Polio reappeared in Syria after a 15-year absence and continues to persist in Pakistan, Afghanistan, parts of Africa, and Iraq. It is particularly concerning in war-torn areas, where even with vaccines are available, people are difficult to reach, or people refuse vaccination. Fortunately, we have a much stronger public health system with partners around the world pitching in to eradicate diseases.

Suggested Reading

Gaynes, *Germ Theory*.

McNeill, *Plagues and Peoples*.

Oshinsky, *Polio*.

Sherman, *Twelve Diseases That Changed Our World*.

Questions to Consider

1. What do you think has been the greatest discovery in medicine since Hippocrates? Why?

2. What do you think historians will write about the current era of infectious diseases? Will it be as interesting as diseases of the past?

Bacteria: Heroes and Villains

Lecture 2

The term "microbes" is a general term for organisms usually too small to be seen by the naked eye. In the human body, these include bacteria, viruses, yeast, protozoa, and a bunch of germs that lie in between these categories. In this lecture, you will learn about some of the essential features of bacteria. You will discover how bacteria can be advantageous, hostile, or simply innocent bystanders. In addition, you will learn about their anatomy and functioning. Furthermore, you will explore how they can cause disease and how they can adapt to make themselves elusive to our immune system.

The Basics of Bacteria

- Bacteria are everywhere. They are very small, usually less than 2 microns in size. For comparison, the width of a human hair is about 75 microns. Bacteria are single-celled organisms that contain the barest essential elements for staying alive and reproducing. These are a chromosome, ribosomes, cytoplasm, and an outer membrane.

- Bacteria are a simple form of life known as prokaryotes. In the center is the genetic code material known as deoxyribonucleic acid (DNA), which is bundled into a single central structure known as a chromosome. DNA encodes for a specific sequence of building blocks known as amino acids, which are combined into proteins in the ribosome structure of the cell. Proteins are subsequently used to control cellular function. There is a membrane around the outside to contain internal fluid, otherwise known as cytoplasm.

- More complex microorganisms contain eukaryotic cells, which have a nucleus that contains multiple strands of DNA organized into multiple chromosomes. They also have more complex internal structures, such as mitochondria, which produce internal energy. Eukaryotic cells utilize more formal membrane structures, such as a nuclear membrane, to contain the DNA. The simplest one-cell

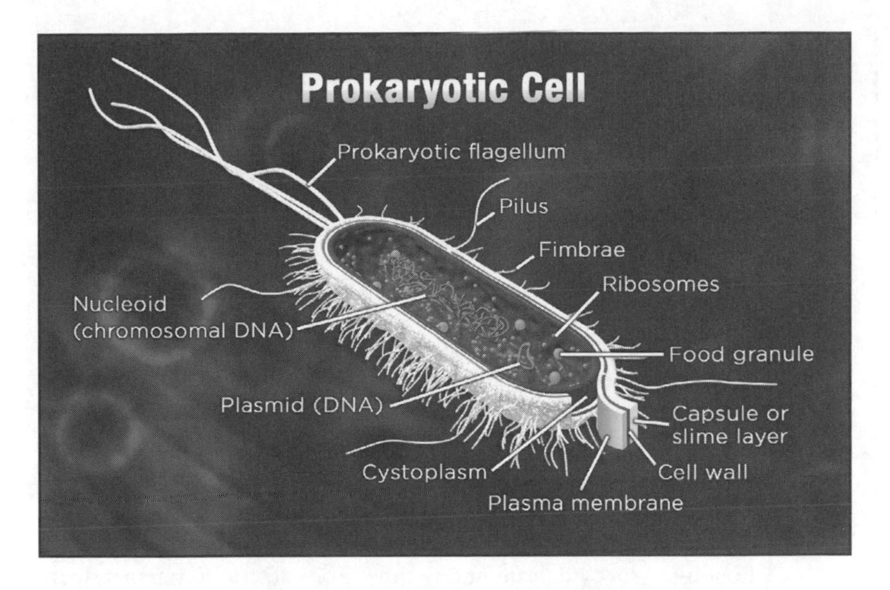

eukaryote is a protozoa called a paramecium. Other examples of multicellular eukaryotes include fungi, plants, and animals.

- Prokaryotic bacterial reproduction is under the control of the genetic code, DNA, wrapped together in an organized giant loop called a chromosome. Because bacteria multiply so rapidly, often in minutes, by a process known as binary fission, the repeat replication of DNA is prone to errors. Hence, genetic mutations can occur that either lead to either a survival advantage or disadvantage.

- DNA replication is controlled by an enzyme protein known as DNA polymerase. It is a prime target for antibiotics, because the antibiotic's goal is to halt DNA replication. Some DNA may not be in the center of the cell but instead may be located in the cytoplasm, forming circles of DNA known as plasmids. Plasmid DNA may also be transferred from one bacterium to another through various mechanisms when bacteria touch one another.

- Conjugation is one of these means. When this happens, genetic characteristics among bacteria are shared. This is important in the development of bacteria that are resistant to multiple antibiotics, or for other evolutionary traits that support their survival.

- Synthesis of cellular proteins, such as enzymes or toxins, is under the control of DNA, acting through the ribosomes, which combine amino acid building blocks in the cytoplasm. The ribosome is also an excellent target for antibiotics because they can interfere with protein synthesis.

- Enzymes are responsible for controlling all the ongoing work in a cell. Enzymes are chemical-reaction machines, either breaking molecules apart or putting molecules together. This is how a cell functions from minute to minute. Another enzyme function is to link together amino acid building blocks to form a protein.

- A bacterium may have more than 1,000 different types of enzymes floating in its cytoplasm at any time. For bacteria to interact, there are special structures called fimbriae and pili on the surface that can help them attach to other bacterium, or human cells.

Good Bacteria

- Bacterial interactions with humans can be divided into three general categories. First, some germs are good bacteria and help us directly, such as assisting in food digestion. Second, some germs are known as commensal bacteria, which live happily with other bacteria without causing us harm. Third, some bacteria are harmful and are known as pathogenic.

- What roles do the good bacteria play in some of our organ systems? For example, the job of the bacteria in the intestines is to break down nutrients, such as sugars and fats, which humans otherwise could not digest. Most of these gut bacteria do not like the oxygen in the air and are known as anaerobes, meaning that they favor growth in an environment with little or no oxygen.

- Besides aiding in digestion, some gut bacteria also synthesize certain vitamins and aid the immune system. More specifically,

Escherichia coli, or *E. coli*, is the most common bacterium that usually lives in the last part our intestine, the colon. Unlike others, this germ happens to like oxygen, so it's known as an aerobic bacterium. *E coli* has been extensively studied and is probably the best-understood bacterium.

- *E. coli* is usually associated with something bad, such as traveler's diarrhea, but this germ can be both good and bad. Its good role is to synthesize vitamin K, which is essential for normal blood clotting. When patients are receiving antibiotics, the antibiotics can kill their good *E. coli* as innocent bystanders and alter clotting function.

- In recent years, good bacteria have been in the news, and there is a renewed interest in our own bacteria, known as the human microbiome. Thanks to the Human Microbiome Project, launched in 2007, scientists are learning about the influence of microbes on physiology, human development, immunity, and nutrition. Five microbiome body sites are being studied: the nose, mouth, intestines, vagina, and skin.

Bad Bacteria

- A pathogen is any germ that can cause damage and disease via its interaction with a host. Humans often harbor bacteria with pathogenic potential on our skin or in our mouth. But unless the right circumstances occur that lead to invasion, there usually are no consequences for simple colonization by these pathogenic bacteria. Instead, a person may serve as a carrier to transmit disease to others.

- What are some characteristics that make bacteria pathogenic and cause human disease? Bacteria have the ability to create toxins, which are chemical poisons that interfere with cell function; digest normal human enzymes; evade infection-fighting white blood cells and immune clearance; produce protective capsules, or "slime material," so they can't be swallowed by white blood cells; and adapt DNA that can encode for antibiotic resistance.

- Even good bacteria in the wrong place can cause infections. The microbes that inhabit the skin and mucous membranes, such as the mouth, are known as normal flora or normal microbiota. They play a part in the normal, healthy human physiology—unless they become too populous or inhabit places in the body that they don't belong, such as the bloodstream.

- Another important concept is that there are some anatomical sites within the body that are normally sterile. These include, for example, the areas around the brain and spinal cord as well as the lower portions of the lungs. When bacteria invade these normally sterile spaces, they usually will produce disease and, hence, become pathogenic. For example, bacteria in the spinal fluid will cause bacterial meningitis.

- How do bacteria invade these sterile areas of the body? There can be any number of entry points for bacteria, such as cuts or breaks in the skin, mucous membranes of the mouth, or even intestines. For example, staphylococcal bacteria can invade a hole in the skin and cause skin abscesses.

Classifying Bacteria

- One of the simplest ways to classify bacteria visually is on the basis of a specific stain: the gram stain. This method is named after the Danish bacteriologist, Hans Gram, who devised the technique in 1882. It is one of the most important staining techniques in microbiology. It is usually the first test performed by the microbiology lab and infectious disease specialists in the identification of bacteria.

- The gram stain procedure distinguishes between gram-positive, or violet-colored, bacteria and gram-negative, or red-colored, bacteria. It has three steps: staining with violet dye, decoloring with acetone or alcohol, and counterstaining with safranine, which is a red dye.

- Gram-positive bacteria stain purple due to the presence of a specific sugar layer in their cell membrane, which retains the crystal violet stain and is not washed out by alcohol. Gram-negative bacteria, on the other hand, stain pink, because they have a thinner sugar wall, which allows the crystal violet dye to get washed out during the decoloring process with alcohol. Restaining with a safranine dye results in a red color.

Virulence Factors

- The DPT vaccine contains three bacteria that produce dangerous toxins: *Corynebacterium diphtheria*, *Bordetella pertussis*, and *Clostridium tetani*. *Corynebacterium diphtheria* is gram-positive staining and aerobic and has a rodlike shape.

- *Corynebacterium diphtheria* is a germ that is not normally found in the back of the throat, but before the DPT vaccine was developed, this germ sometimes found its way to the back of the throat and into the nose. When this happened, it caused a sore throat, fever, and swollen glands. But the classic sign of diphtheria disease is a sheet of thick, gray material covering the back of the throat, blocking the airway, and causing difficulty breathing.

- Diphtheria infections are somewhat unusual, because the bacteria only invade the surface cells of the throat. However, the protein toxin produced spreads through the circulation and nonspecifically attacks other cells of the body.

- Severe infection with diphtheria toxin can cause death by interrupting the function of essential organs such as the heart, kidneys, liver, and lungs—blocking all protein synthesis in affected cells by interfering with a key enzyme in the ribosomes.

- How does this bacterium enhance its own survival? When a person coughs or sneezes, the germs are spread through tiny droplets into the air, where they can infect others within an eight-foot range. They can also spread from the mucus on a used tissue or from silverware that's been in an infected person's mouth.

- In the United States, due to the efficacy of the DPT vaccine, there is rarely a case of diphtheria anymore. Russia and Eastern Europe have not been as fortunate, where there are thousands of cases, due to low rates of vaccination.

- *Bordetella pertussis*, which causes the illness whooping cough, is caused by an extremely contagious germ through respiratory droplets. After the germ settles in the respiratory tract, the bacterium uses several toxins to bind and destroy the epithelial, or surface lining, cells. The pertussis toxin enters cells and interferes with communication between cells. Also, it releases a throat cytotoxin, which causes the destruction of the hairs, known as cilia, in the epithelial cell layer. Cilia are responsible for keeping our airways free from bad bacteria.

- *Clostridium tetani*, a bacterium that can generally be found in the soil everywhere, causes tetanus, an illness that leads to spasms of all the muscles of the body. One hallmark of the disease is the jaw of the mouth getting stuck, giving the illness the nickname "lockjaw." Spores, which are a dried-out, dormant form of the bacterium, can survive in the soil for many years. When the spores are exposed to a favorable environment, such as water and sugar, the bacterium can become active again.

- In addition to toxin production, another deadly virulence factor of gram-negative bacteria is endotoxin. With the infamous plague bacteria *Yersinia pestis*, the outer gram-negative cellular membrane also contains a special compound known as lipopolysaccharide (LPS). LPS contains a compound known as lipid A, which is extremely toxic to humans and forms the basis of endotoxin. When bacterial cells are broken apart by our immune system, or by antibiotics, fragments of the cell membrane containing lipid A are released into the bloodstream, releasing endotoxin. This can trigger a deadly cascade of events known as the sepsis syndrome, more commonly known as blood poisoning.

- Another factor that helps bacteria escape the immune system is thick capsules that are protective barriers made of sugars outside the cell membranes. They enable bacteria to be more evasive, because white blood cells, which are part of our immune system, are subsequently unable to swallow the germs.

- Next, the biofilm, which is an extracellular sugar network that forms a scaffolding around the bacteria (basically a slime layer), allows bacteria to bind to artificial devices such as plastic intravenous catheters or artificial joints. The germs go into hibernation, and the biofilm protects the germs from the immune system.

- Finally, some bacteria may be swallowed by our white blood cells but yet manage to survive inside these cells unharmed. These bacteria inhibit specific killing mechanisms and are thus safe from our immune defenses.

Suggested Reading

Blaser, *Missing Microbes*.

Gladwin and Trattler, *Clinical Microbiology Made Ridiculously Simple*.

Leavitt, *Typhoid Mary*.

Margulis and Sagan, *Microcosmos*.

Questions to Consider

1. What is the importance of the human bacterial microbiome to your personal health?

2. Whooping cough, diphtheria, and tetanus germs can be deadly in unvaccinated populations around the world. What is your view on forced vaccination of populations to control disease?

Viruses: Hijackers of Your Body's Cells

Lecture 3

In this lecture, you will learn all about the world of viruses, along with several germs that lie between the categories of bacteria and viruses. Specifically, you will learn about the herpes simplex virus types 1 and 2; a variant of normal bacteria known as a spirochete, which causes Lyme disease and syphilis; and rickettsia, which is a hybrid between a bacterium and a virus, causing an illness known as typhus. You will also learn about the historical significance of some of these infamous viruses.

Viruses

- The first virus was conceptually isolated in 1895, when laboratory filters that were too small to allow bacteria to pass were used. The smaller virus particles passed through the filter and were identified as the tobacco mosaic virus, typically found on tobacco and tomato plants. Because viruses are at least 100 times smaller than bacteria, they can't be seen under the light microscope. They were first seen in 1931, when the electron microscope was invented.

- Viruses are life-forms whose genetic material, either DNA or RNA, replicates inside living cells using the other cell's synthetic machinery. This leads to the synthesis of components of the virus that are subsequently reassembled and then transferred to either other living host cells or sometimes into the environment.

- Viruses have no capacity for independent protein synthesis or for generation of their own energy supplies. They have no cell wall or nucleus. They reproduce by assembly of various viral pieces and not by growth and division like bacteria do. They are totally dependent on the host cell for survival.

- There are several steps in a viral replication, including attachment to a cell, entry inside the cell, early genetic expression, DNA or

RNA replication, late genetic expression, assembly of new viruses, and release of daughter viruses from the cell.

- First, the virus attaches to the host cell. Attachment involves two minimum components: a virus attachment complex and cellular receptors for the virus. Some cellular receptors are proteins, such as for HIV, while others are sugar receptors, such as sialic acid for influenza.

- Next, the virus enters the cells. The virus crosses the cell membranes either by melting and merging with the cell membrane or by being swallowed by the cell. Then, viruses utilize one of three unique patterns of replication, depending on which genetic material they possess: DNA, RNA, or RNA retrovirus.
    - For DNA viruses, its DNA must enter the host cell's nucleus to replicate. The DNA polymerase enzyme of the host cell is hijacked for viral DNA replication.

    - RNA is foreign genetic material to human cells, because humans do not have RNA. Therefore, the first step for RNA virus replication is to trick the host cells to produce an RNA polymerase, which subsequently allows the RNA virus to be replicated.

    - The third type of replication involves retroviruses—such as human immunodeficiency virus (HIV)—which have a unique

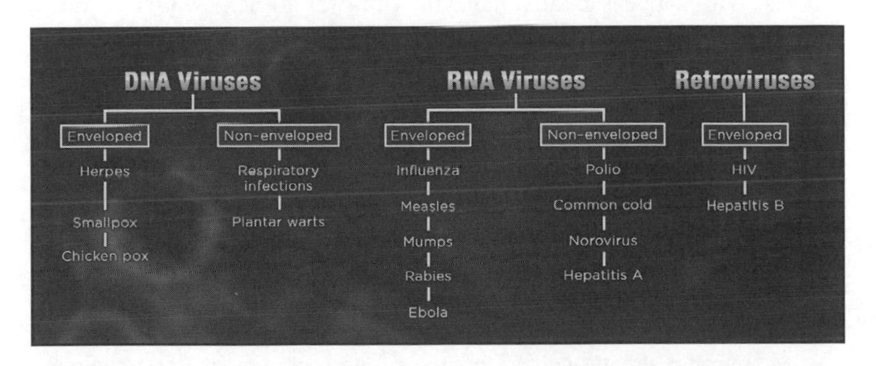

mechanism of replication. A retrovirus possesses one copy of a single-stranded RNA. It also carries with it a unique enzyme known as reverse transcriptase. Shortly after cell entry, the single RNA strand is copied into a double-stranded DNA spiral helix, the reverse of the normal replication process. Retroviruses also like to integrate their genetic material into the host cell with a different retrovirus enzyme called integrase. The host cell then treats the foreign viral DNA as part of its own genome. This new DNA infection will persist indefinitely.

- When viruses replicate, they do so in a rapid exponential fashion, which generates millions of new virus particles. Even more so than for bacteria, this is significant because random genetic mutations are more frequent than with bacteria and can lead to the "survival of the fittest" viruses. This is particularly important for targeting antiviral therapy for HIV; combinations of medications need to be taken to help prevent the emergence of this viral resistance.

- After the virus DNA or RNA replicates in a host cell, it directs the cell to help the virus package itself in the cytoplasm, and then the virus breaks free from the host cell either into neighboring cells or often into the bloodstream. Viral infections can be classified as either localized, where the virus remains at the site of entry, or body-wide, otherwise known as disseminated.

- What happens to the cell that the virus was in? Some viral infections, such as Ebola, result in complete host cell shutdown, leading to cell death. Other viruses may selectively inhibit a specific host cell function, allowing the cell to survive but in a damaged form. If the cells survive in a damaged condition, subsequent bacterial infection, known as a superinfection, can occur several days later. This is a common mechanism of disease for respiratory viruses, which may lead to secondary bacterial ear or sinus infections, or even bacterial pneumonia.

- Viruses are classified by their genetic material as DNA, RNA, or retroviruses as well as by their outer component—as enveloped or non-enveloped. Because viruses are structurally completely different than bacteria, no antibiotics will work in preventing virus replication. Therefore, getting antibiotics for a bad cold will not help you recover faster. Antiviral medications exist, but there are not many when compared with antibiotics. This is why vaccination against viral illnesses is important.

- Sneezing and coughing are easy ways for germs to spread, but larger droplets settle quickly from the air and are not contagious. Viruses are more likely to spread via wet secretions that contaminate surfaces in the environment. Many of these viruses can survive up to four days on solid surfaces.

The Family of Herpes Viruses

- The herpes virus family has 100 members, but there are 4 main ones of human significance: herpes simplex virus type 1 (HSV-1) and 2 (HSV-2); Epstein-Barr virus, which is responsible for infectious mononucleosis; varicella-zoster virus, which is responsible for chicken pox and shingles; and cytomegalovirus, which is responsible for some newborn infections and even birth defects.

- All the herpes viruses can not only cause an acute infection, but they also are never eliminated from our bodies and exist in a dormant, or hibernating, state throughout our lives. HSV-1, while causing fever blisters, can also cause clinical disease in a wide variety of other anatomic locations. HSV-2 is usually known as genital herpes.

- During a person's first exposure to the virus, otherwise known as primary infection, introduction—sometimes called inoculation—of herpes at mucosal surfaces, or moist skin sites, permits entry of the virus through the top layers of the skin. Next, the virus invades the closest nerve endings.

- Local symptoms begin within a few days, with the appearance of multiple blister-type lesions superimposed on a red base. Sores in the mouth and a severe sore throat with blisters are frequent manifestations of primary HSV-1 infection, whereas so-called fever blisters are the most frequent sign of recurrent disease.

- A primary infection with herpes, either oral or genital, is usually associated with body-wide flulike symptoms, along with fever and malaise. The blisters are painful and last for about 10 days. Vesicles are usually grouped in a single anatomic site; however, if one touches the sores, they can be spread to other body locations.

- Most primary herpes infections are asymptomatic, meaning that there are no symptoms. This has tremendous implications for disease transmission, because herpes virus can be shed without clinical signs of disease and can lead to stealthy transmission via contact with secretions.

Syphilis

- Spirochetes have many of the same characteristics as bacteria but are different enough biologically that they don't stain with the routine gram stain. Two common examples are the *Borrelia burgdorferi*, which is the Lyme disease germ, and *Treponema pallidum*, which is the syphilis germ.

- Syphilis is a sexually transmitted disease. The germ that causes syphilis, *Treponenum pallidum*, is a thin spirochete that can survive only briefly outside the human body. Infection is divided into three stages.
    - The primary stage appears as one or more painless, firm, red ulcers called chancres of the skin at the site of inoculation. Ulcers most commonly occur on the genitals an average of three weeks after exposure and heal spontaneously.

    - The secondary stage is characterized by a rash, flulike symptoms, and generalized body-wide lymph node enlargement that appear within a few months. This stage also resolves spontaneously without treatment, leaving the infected person asymptomatic.

- The third stage of infection, if untreated, occurs 15 to 30 years after the initial infection and can include unusual and bizarre manifestations of the body, such as dementia of the brain or ruptured blood vessels leading to death.

- Today, there are still about 12 million cases of syphilis around the world. Its incidence is also related to the incidence of HIV, and there is a two to five percent chance of being infected with both, because the primary means of transmission is by sexual intercourse.

- A hot debate has been going on for years regarding the origin of syphilis. The disease seemed to have originated in a non-sexually-related form, often seen in children, then adapted to a venereal disease, which means it is primarily associated with sexual intercourse, due to changes in behaviors of people at a certain time in history and likely as a means of enhancing its own survival.

- Another historical debate is whether syphilis's origin was in the Old World or New World—specifically, before Columbus sailed to America or after he returned to Europe. Researchers have speculated for years that Christopher Columbus's voyage brought not only news of a new world but also syphilis from the Americas. A comprehensive study done by Emory University in 2011 seems to confirm that it came aboard the *Niña*, the only ship to make it back to Spain.

- Once syphilis arrived in Europe, it took only five years to become an epidemic. Then, it quickly spread throughout the Old World—and then throughout Asia, and to every continent except Antarctica. It wasn't until four centuries later that the specific disease-causing spirochete germ was identified in 1905.

- Regardless of its origin, syphilis was a devastating disease that killed many thousands of people all over the world. In the United States, the incidence of syphilis, which had been declining into the 21st century, is beginning to rise. This is predominately due to a change in some sexual values.

Typhus

- Rickettsias are singled-celled, non-virus, non-bacterial germs that have gram-negative bacterial structural characteristics but are intracellular rod-shaped parasites, which, like viruses, must live inside cells to survive. So, they are a sort of hybrid between a bacteria and a virus.

- Rickettsias are usually transmitted by blood-sucking parasites, such as fleas, lice, and ticks. Rickettsias live in the parasite's intestines, but the parasite does not develop any disease. Rather, rickettsias are transmitted by parasite excrement or mouthparts.

- This germ was named after Howard Ricketts, an American pathologist who ironically died after identifying typhus as a rickettsial disease. (Note that typhus should not be confused with typhoid, which is a disease caused by salmonella bacteria.) Other rickettsial diseases include trench fever, which was common in WWI and is transmitted by rat fleas, and Rocky Mountain spotted fever, which is transmitted by ticks.

- Typhus in its normal epidemic form is caused by *Rickettsia prowazekii*. It is a deadly louse-borne disease with a distinctive rash that killed hundreds of thousands of soldiers. When Napoleon retreated from Moscow in 1812, more French soldiers died of typhus than were killed by the Russians. This trend of typhus helping to determine the outcome of wars carried over to WWI and WWII.

- Epidemic typhus is now a rare disease. However, thousands of cases occurred in Burundi in Southeast Africa in association with civil war during the 1990s; body louse infestation preceded the outbreaks. This was also called jail fever, and it epitomizes the problems with crowding and lack of hygiene.

- How do rickettsias cause disease in humans? The clinical manifestations are due to the ability of the rickettsias to multiply inside the endothelial cells, the first layer of cells lining the small blood vessels. These infected cells detach from the blood vessels and block blood circulation, eventually leading to deprivation of oxygen in tissues and cell destruction. This is also how U.S. citizens die of Rocky Mountain spotted fever, which can cause rapid death.

Suggested Reading

Booss and August, *To Catch a Virus*.

Crawford, *The Invisible Enemy*.

Gladwin and Trattler, *Clinical Microbiology Made Ridiculously Simple*.

Harper and Meyer, *Of Mice, Men and Microbes*.

Zimmer, *A Planet of Viruses*.

Questions to Consider

1. Of bacteria, viruses, and in-between germs, which category do you think will be most problematic in the future?

2. Do you think your community should do more in terms of educational efforts regarding influenza and the spread of disease?

Moldy Menaces and Fungal Diseases

Lecture 4

In this lecture, you will be introduced to another type of microorganism: fungi. Fungi are eukaryotic cells containing a nucleus and many organelles; when compared to bacteria, they are more complicated life-forms that require oxygen to live. As you will learn in this lecture, fungi can cause a wide variety of infections. Although fungal diseases usually don't involve humans, they can indirectly affect humans. In fact, fungi are capable of devastating crops, animals, and humans in various ways.

Fungal Basics

- Fungi are structurally divided into yeasts (similar to the yeast used in baking bread) and molds (the green circles on moldy pieces of bread or old blocks of cheese). Molds are composed of many hyphal elements. Hyphae are threadlike, branching tubules composed of fungal cells attached end to end.

- Most fungi are either yeasts or molds. However, there are some fungi that are dimorphic, meaning that they exist in one shape in the human body and a different shape on laboratory culture media. Yeasts are unicellular growth forms of fungi. These cells can appear spherical to elliptical, and they reproduce by budding. The reproducing bodies of molds are spores.

- The cell membranes of fungi are also more complex than those of bacteria. The outer cell contains a building block known as ergosterol, which is similar in structure to cholesterol, which is in the structure of human membranes. Some antifungal medications may have side effects that are associated with the structural similarity between ergosterol and cholesterol.

- Fungal infections are generally categorized by the depth of the invasion into the human body: surface-based skin infections, infections underneath the skin, body-wide infections associated

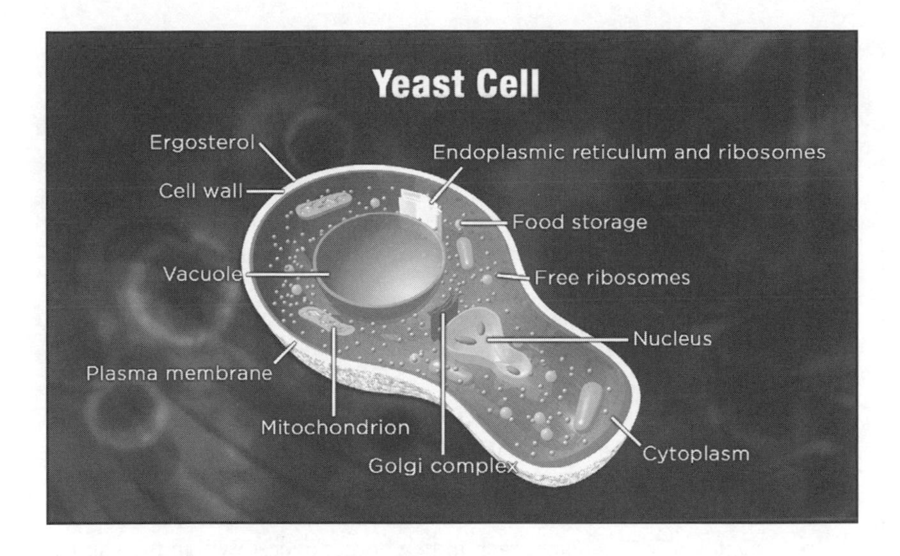

with specific geographic areas, and infections in patients with compromised immune systems.

Fungal Infections

- Fungal infections of the skin surfaces, hair, and nails are known as dermatophytes. These fungi live in the dead, outside layers of the skin, hair, and nails. Keratin is the primary structural protein of these body components. Dermatophytes secrete an enzyme, keratinase, which partially digests layers of these body components.

- The disruption of keratin causes loss of hair, scaling of the skin, and crumbling of the nails. When the nails are involved, the term is known as onychomycosis. This leads to thickened, discolored, and brittle nails. Fungal nail infections become more prevalent as we age, with about half of adults being affected by age 70.

- Superficial fungal infections are nicknamed "tinea." Tinea corporis forms a ring shape with a red raised border and is known as ringworm. When these dermatophytes involve the scalp, they are known as tinea capitis. When they involve the foot, they are known as tinea pedis and cause athlete's foot, which results in the cracking and peeling of skin between the toes.

- Moving deeper into the skin, subcutaneous fungal infections usually enter the body following injury to the skin rather than a digestive enzyme. They usually remain localized to the tissues just underneath the top layer of the skin or spread to local lymph nodes.

- An important yeast that can cause either a superficial or subcutaneous fungal infection is known as *Candida albicans*. Candida species, like bacteria, are part of the body's normal microbiota. When antibiotics can kill the bacteria but not the yeast, candida can take advantage of the lack of bacteria and expand their growth without competition.

- Candida causes diaper rash in newborns; overgrowth in the vaginal area after antibiotics, leading to a white discharge; or a white pattern in the mouth known as oral thrush, which is seen after antibiotic therapy. Candida can also be involved in body-wide infections in patients who are hospitalized and subjected to antibiotic therapy and invasive medical devices, such as intravenous catheters.

- The most common fungal infections that cause systemic, or body-wide, disease in humans are histoplasmosis, blastomycosis, and coccidioidomycosis. All three are dimorphic fungi, growing as mold in the laboratory and as yeast in the human body.

- What is unique about these three fungal diseases is that they characteristically inhabit unique geographic areas of the United States and hence are known as endemic mycoses. Histoplasmosis and blastomycosis are commonly found in the drainage area of the Mississippi River Valley area, but isolated cases of both diseases may occur in other parts of the country. Coccidioidomycosis is unique to the Southwestern United States, including Arizona, New Mexico, and Southern California.

- All three endemic mycoses have one of three clinical presentations. The majority of cases are asymptomatic—or, worse, a mild respiratory infection that generally does not get reported, nor even lead to a medical visit. When a more significant load of fungal spores is inhaled, this will lead to pneumonia.

- Usually, with a normal immune system, the body will recover without specific antifungal therapy. However, now that antifungal therapy is more readily available, these pneumonias can be treated and resolved sooner with medications. On rare occasions, these fungal diseases can spread outside the lung throughout the body, including to the brain, liver, and spleen. The disease is labeled as "disseminated."

- Histoplasmosis outbreaks are notorious for occurring after common exposures, such as cleaning a chicken coop, clearing a bird roost, demolishing an old building, or exploring a cave where bat guano is abundant. The mold especially likes to live in the soil, where bird or bat droppings provide extra nutrients to support its growth.

Other Fungal Infections

- *Cryptococcus neoformans* is a yeast that is found in the soil throughout the United States and, when inhaled by patients with compromised immune systems, can lead to pneumonia and a serious infection around the brain and spinal cord known as fungal meningitis. Cryptococcus has a very thick-walled, sugar-based capsule, which prevents white blood cells from attacking and destroying the yeast. Hence, aggressive antifungal therapy is required to successfully treat this dangerous and often life-threatening condition.

- A multistate outbreak of fungal meningitis and infectious arthritis was detected in the Eastern United States in late September of 2012. More than 700 patients who had received steroid injections produced at a single pharmaceutical compounding center developed meningitis or spinal infections, and more than 30 patients who received injections into joints, such as the knees, of the same steroid developed infections.

- *Ex-sero-hilum* species, a brown-black fungus, was the cause. The injections were being given for pain, because steroids reduce inflammation and pain by shutting down the body's immune response at the site of injection. The average time from injection to the beginning of symptoms was 18 days.

- Further epidemiologic investigation revealed that the risk of infection was associated with specific batches of the steroid and with older vials. Also, the more injections individuals received and the larger the volume of steroids, the greater the risk of infection.

- The Tennessee Department of Health sounded the alarm based on a telephone call from an alert clinician treating a patient with this unusual form of meningitis. With information rapidly communicated from Tennessee, the Centers for Disease Control and Prevention reached out to state and local health departments and took collective action. Within days, the source of the outbreak was identified, and a massive effort was undertaken to identify and contact the nearly 14,000 potentially exposed patients and their physicians across 23 states.

- Voriconazole, an antifungal medication, was used to treat most patients, but some were also treated with a special, more dangerous antifungal medication, amphotericin B. Because amphotericin does not distinguish well between ergosterol and cholesterol in cell membranes, serious side effects, such as kidney failure, occurred. Unfortunately, there were many deaths and many patients left with long-term disabilities from this outbreak.

Environmental Mold

- In spite of the "clean" air in your home, there are actually thousands of fungal mold spores that are floating around outside, invisible in the air. Normally, our immune system is sufficiently strong so that occasional spores that land in our lungs do not cause infection.

- In patients with compromised immune systems, these spores can enter the lung and cause an established fungal infection of the lung. Aspergillus is the most common mold to cause infection in immune-compromised patients. This is a significant problem with transplant recipients—up to five percent of transplant patients may die from invasive fungal infections when Aspergillus is inhaled in the lung and the immune system cannot compensate.

- What would happen, even with a normal immune system, if the air were filled with a large number of fungal mold spores? Would we get sick? Some individuals may manifest non-life-threatening yet annoying allergic symptoms from mold, similar to hay-fever allergies. Those already with allergies may notice the allergies being more severe.

- Sometimes, concerns are raised regarding mold overgrowth in buildings producing "toxins" causing so-called sick building syndrome, or mold illness in the home environment from toxins. The term "toxic mold" is not a real clinical disease entity. The actual mold is usually not directly toxic, and by and large, having your household duct system routinely cleaned is an unnecessary expense. Allergy sufferers may find this individually useful.

Antifungal Medications

- A variety of antifungal medications have been developed to treat various fungal conditions. Some of these medications are topical. For example, gentian violet was used for treatment of ringworm. This is rarely used today, because other topical medications are usually effective for superficial fungal infections. However, treatment of fungal nail infections presents an extreme challenge. There is a low rate—only 5 to 10 percent—of long-term success, so gentian violet is still used for this condition.

- The prototype antifungal medications are known as azole drugs. They interrupt the cell wall synthesis in fungi, blocking ergosterol production and leading to the incomplete synthesis of the cell wall. Because fungi do not replicate as quickly as bacteria and have a slower growth metabolism, antifungal therapy needs to be continued for longer than antibiotics.

- Two other antifungal drugs used for systemic infections include the echinocandin medications and amphotericin. Echinocandins disrupt the cross-linking of the fungal cell wall. Amphotericin directly attacks the fungal cell wall, leading to alterations in the permeability of the wall and subsequent fungal cell death.

Suggested Reading

Gladwin and Trattler, *Clinical Microbiology Made Ridiculously Simple*.

Kauffman, Pappas, Sobel, and Dismukes, *Essentials of Clinical Mycology*.

Questions to Consider

1. Have you ever swept or used a blower to clean out a garage or barn where animals have been? What precautions should you take when coming into contact with air and dust that may contain airborne germs?

2. Do you live in an area of the United States where outdoor recreational activity, or even home renovation, could make you susceptible to contracting a fungal disease?

Milestones in Infectious Disease History

Lecture 5

Where would we be without inventors and innovators that brought to life inventions and discoveries that are the foundations of modern medicine? In this lecture, you will be introduced to some of the people who have helped develop infectious disease tools to identify different microorganisms in the effort to control them. You will learn about some of the most important individuals and their contributions to infectious diseases and how their scientific breakthroughs may have changed the course of history.

Hippocrates

- Hippocrates, often deemed the father of modern medicine, was a 5th-century Greek physician who founded the Hippocratic School of Medicine, a college that at the time revolutionized the understanding of medicine in ancient Greece. He taught medical students at the school, focusing on the skills necessary to make detailed clinical observations, diagnoses, and prognoses.

- In Greek medicine, doctors believed that people's constitutional makeup predisposed them to certain diseases. The human constitution could be broken down into four humors, or vital fluids. The humors were known as the four universal elements: earth, air, fire, and water.

- In this ancient scheme, earth is linked to black bile, a sediment of blood that is important in metabolism, bone formation, and clotting; water is linked to phlegm, which lubricates and nourishes the body; fire is linked to yellow bile, which affects the intestinal system and the digestion and processing of fats and cholesterol; and air, which is linked to red blood cells and is thought to be the purest humor because it is essential for vitality and growth. If one of these humors was out of balance, it was believed that it led to illness and disease.

- In addition, each humor was associated with a particular season and psychological temperament. For example, blood, or spring, was associated with optimism and well-being. Hippocrates believed that physical health and individual personalities were parts of your whole health.

- The negative characteristics of the humors were thought to come out only when they were excessive or aggravated by imbalances. An excess in one humor led to the practice of bloodletting, which was used to expel harmful surpluses of one of the humors. This theory also began the practice of using medicinal leeches.

- One of Hippocrates's most important contributions to infectious diseases is that he was the first to recognize that specific diseases come from unique causes. Greek society at the time believed that disease was the result of miasma (bad air) or was due to superstitions or works of the gods as punishments.

- Because the government forbade the dissection of bodies, it was difficult to accurately study disease. Hippocrates's beliefs went against those of the government, and he was imprisoned for 20 years. Fortunately, during his imprisonment, he was able to write important medical books, such as *The Complicated Body*, that set a course for the future of modern medicine.

The Beginning of the Study of Infectious Disease

- As early as the 13th century, special lenses that magnified images formed a primitive microscope. One of the most important events during the 1600s was the development of the modern light microscope to identify specific germs. Although combining lenses to attempt to increase magnification had been attempted in the 1600s, they were difficult to build and could only enhance objects by 20 to 30 times.

- Anton van Leeuwenhoek, considered to be the father of microbiology, constructed microscopes and used them to discover bacteria in 1674. He was the first to identify single-celled organisms, as well as muscle fibers and blood flow through capillaries.

- Robert Hooke, designated the English father of microscopy, is famous for his book *Micrographia*, which contains fantastic copperplate engravings of his findings. He was the first to use the term "cell" to describe what he saw, as he looked at slices of cork through his microscope that were divided into individual spaces. He confirmed Leeuwenhoek's discoveries and improved on the microscope's design.

Smallpox

- One of modern medicine's true triumphs has been smallpox's subsequent eradication. The cause of smallpox is the variola virus. The disease became widespread in Europe and Asia, killing half a million Europeans yearly at the turn of the 19th century, with more than 80 percent of these being children.

- Smallpox enters the body through infectious particles contacting the mucous membranes, or via the respiratory system by inhalation of droplets. From its initial site of invasion, it spreads locally to lymph nodes and then jumps into the bloodstream, where it then can invade other major organs. The pox on the skin is the visual clue of the internal disease.

- Colonization of the New World carried smallpox to the Americas. Ironically, it played a major role in the conquest of Mexico and Peru, as well as the European settlement of North America. Many of the indigenous Native American populations, whose immune systems had never previously been exposed to the virus, couldn't fight the disease and died.

- As late as the 20th century, there were millions of worldwide deaths from smallpox. The World Health Organization (WHO) estimated that as recently as 1967, 15 million people contracted smallpox and 2 million died of it that year. In order to reduce the risk of smallpox, an ingenious preventive inoculation called variolation was devised as early as the 10th century in Asia.

- Individuals were deliberately infected with smallpox by blowing dried smallpox scabs into the nose of an individual. These individuals usually contracted a mild form of smallpox, leaving them immune. Only one or two percent of these patients died, compared to a 30-percent mortality rate for others dying from smallpox without variolation prevention.

- In 1700, this procedure was being widely used in India, Africa, and the Ottoman Empire. But smallpox was still a serious disease with no treatment. Therefore, developing a more scientific vaccination for prevention was a world health-care priority.

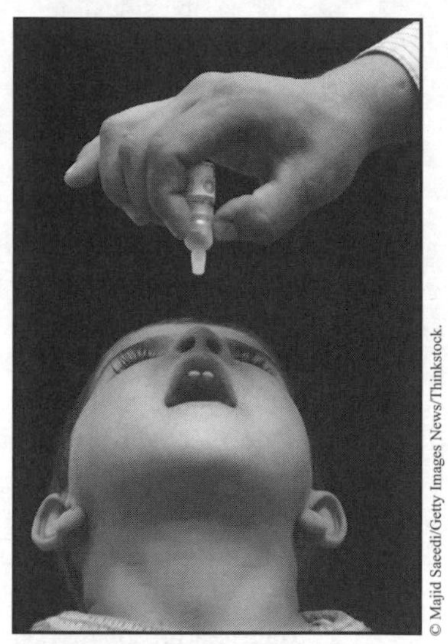

Vaccines administered in childhood can prevent the child from becoming infected with certain diseases.

- A more traditional type of smallpox immunization was developed in 1796 by Edward Jenner, an English physician. Even though he was unaware that smallpox was caused by a virus, he discovered that immunity to smallpox could be conveyed by inoculating a person with material from a cowpox lesion, a poxvirus in the same family. He called the material "vaccine." The smallpox vaccine is no longer a cowpox derivative like Jenner's. Instead, it is a live vaccine derived from a similar poxvirus—the vaccinia virus.

- The last case of smallpox in the United States was in 1949, but in 1967, the disease was still endemic in 31 countries. Because the incubation period for smallpox is relatively long, 7 to 17 days, and quarantine can be effective in halting transmission, smallpox was a prime candidate for worldwide eradication.

- The WHO worked hard over the next 10 years to eradicate the disease, and the last naturally occurring smallpox case in the world was in Somalia in 1977. In 1980, the world was declared free of smallpox. Except for laboratory stockpiles, smallpox has been eliminated. However, there is heightened concern since 9/11 that the virus might be used as an agent of bioterrorism, and contingency plans are in place from governments around the world.

Cholera

- Another major infectious disease, which reared its ugly head in Europe beginning in the early 1800s, was cholera, a bacterial disease that followed world trade routes, killing thousands of people in its wake. The symptoms of violent vomiting and diarrhea caused severe dehydration. Cholera victims often died within hours. Fluid losses led to low blood pressure, and alterations in the sodium and potassium content of the blood led to cases of cardiac sudden death.

- During six worldwide pandemics caused by cholera, millions died across all continents. The seventh wave of a pandemic began in South Asia in 1961, spread to Africa in 1971, and then to Central and South America in 1991.

- Cholera is now present in low levels in many countries and still kills thousands yearly. An effective vaccine may finally have been developed and is undergoing continued evaluation. Fortunately, today, death from cholera usually can be prevented by recognizing it early, administering rehydration salts, and replacing fluids, assuming that these resources are available.

- In the 1800s, because the miasma theory of infection was still prevalent, many believed cholera was not contagious, because it didn't seem to easily spread from person to person in those with close contact. An English physician named Dr. John Snow, who did not believe in the miasma theory, hypothesized that the disease was actually being spread through contaminated drinking water. Snow is considered to be the father of contemporary epidemiology, which is the branch of medicine that deals with the incidence, distribution, and possible control of diseases and other factors relating to health.

- Bacteriologist Robert Koch finally identified the specific cholera germ, cholera bacillus, in 1883. Koch was one of the most influential bacteriologists in history. He also proved that microorganisms caused anthrax and tuberculosis. His work was important in proving the germ theory of disease and that diseases were contagious.

- Koch also revolutionized medical epidemiology with his famous four postulates, which have set the standard for proof of infectivity up to the present day. The postulates dictate that a microbe must be found in an animal or person with the disease; isolated and grown in culture; injected into a healthy experimental animal, producing the disease in question; and then recovered from the experimentally diseased animal and shown to be the same pathogen as the original.

Louis Pasteur

- Thanks to Koch, Jenner, and eventually Louis Pasteur, germ theory began to be refined in the mid-1800s. It stated that specific microorganisms are the cause of specific diseases. This theory radically changed the practice of medicine. Scientific proof of this theory was provided by the laboratory research of Louis Pasteur and Robert Koch. Together, their work spurred research that helped identify dangerous germs and develop life-saving treatments.

- Louis Pasteur discovered that beer and milk spoiled because of the rapid multiplication of microbes in these liquids, and this could be prevented through pasteurization. In 1885, Pasteur discovered vaccines for chicken cholera, anthrax, and even the first rabies virus vaccine. Rabies was too small to be seen under any microscope at the time, leading to the concept of smaller organisms, which became known as viruses.

- Perhaps the best thing Pasteur did to revolutionize scientific methodology was to pass on his knowledge to his disciples by creating the Pasteur Institute, encouraging freedom of creative imagination and rigorous scientific experimentation.

- Pasteur worked with another scientist, Charles Chamberland, to invent a device that would enhance the discovery of viruses. In 1884, The Chamberland-Pasteur filter was developed, which completely removed all bacteria from a liquid suspension. By doing this, scientists were able to prove that an unknown infectious substance still remained in the liquid, passing through the smallest-caliber filters. They hence speculated the existence of viruses, even before they were seen.

- In 1898, a Dutch scientist discovered the first virus: the tobacco mosaic virus. By squeezing liquid from an infected tobacco plant and injecting that liquid into a healthy plant, the disease could be transmitted—even though it was put through the special Chamberland-Pasteur filter. Pasteur also implemented methods to improve sanitation, such as cleaning physicians' hands and instruments.

The Electron Microscope

- In the 20th century, there was a need for a new, more powerful microscope: the electron microscope. The invention of this microscope in the 1930s enabled scientists to finally see viruses, which are 100 times smaller than bacteria.

- In the electron microscope, electrons, which are subatomic particles, are accelerated in a vacuum space at short wavelengths. The electrons are directed to a target to form an image on an electron-sensitive photographic plate. Magnification can occur up to 1 million times the original object. Unfortunately, no living specimen can survive the high vacuum pressure and bombardment of electrons, so the microscope cannot show the organism's dynamic life process.

- In the 20th century, many of the worst diseases were found to be caused by specific bacterial or viral pathogens. Vaccines were produced against some organisms, and by the 1950s, antibiotics would begin to cure others. But in the 1960s and 1970s, scientists were potentially becoming overly optimistic about the future conquest of infectious diseases.

- No one could foresee the dynamic nature of infectious diseases, or the serial outbreaks of emerging new infections, such as Legionnaires' disease, Ebola hemorrhagic fever, flesh-eating streptococcal infections, and the HIV or AIDS epidemic.

Suggested Reading

Bud, *Penicillin*.

Crawford, *Deadly Companions*.

Crosby, *The Columbian Exchange*.

De Kruif, *Microbe Hunters*.

Diamond, *Guns, Germs, and Steel*.

Gaynes, *Germ Theory*.

Harrison, *Contagion*.

Sherman, *Twelve Diseases That Changed Our World*.

Questions to Consider

1. What would we know about germs without the invention of the microscope?

2. Why is it that we have been able to eradicate smallpox but still have bacteria like cholera causing significant disease in parts of the world?

Antibiotics: A Modern Miracle Lost?

Lecture 6

Antibiotics have been around since the 1940s and are commonplace today, but we're running out of antibiotics to treat certain illnesses because antibiotic-resistant germs are becoming much more common. This lecture begins by tracing the history of antibiotic development. Then, you will learn about the different classes of antibiotics, as well as their mechanisms of action. In addition, you will be introduced to the increasingly important concern of antibiotic resistance proclaimed by the World Health Organization and the U.S. government. Finally, you will learn how you can contribute to more prudent use of antibiotics.

Historical Perspective on Antibiotics

- In 1888, German scientists observed that the bacterium *Pseudomonas aeruginosa* produced a substance in the test tube known as pyocyanase. Laboratory studies showed that pyocyanase killed dangerous bacteria, such as staphylococcus. However, when it was tried in patients, it was unsuccessful—and even toxic. Pyocyanase was used, however, for nearly 30 more years as a topical skin antibiotic.

- In 1910, Paul Ehrlich, a German chemist, took a different approach. He used a chemical compound called salvarsan, which was an arsenic derivative, to treat syphilis. The drug was toxic, but it represented the first partial success in syphilis treatment. Scientists at the time were striving for a drug that could rid the body of the infecting organism, without harming the patient—a concept we still strive for today.

- In the 1920s, Dr. Alexander Fleming was working in London on a natural chemical from human tears that had antibacterial properties, called lysozyme, which caused bacteria to fall apart. This, too, never succeeded as an antibiotic, but it did show that humans could produce a natural antibacterial substance.

- In 1928, after returning from vacation, Fleming noticed a petri dish with staphylococcal bacteria, whose growth had been inhibited by a mold growing in the adjacent area. He eventually demonstrated that the mold was a penicillium fungus—an unknown substance—produced by the mold that must have traveled across the agar plate to kill bacteria. This substance was henceforth named penicillin. But it would still be another 10 to 15 years before full advantage could be taken of this discovery, with penicillin's first human use in 1941.

Classes of Antibiotics

- There are eight different classes of antibiotics: beta-lactams, sulfonamides, aminoglycosides, chloramphenicol, tetracycline, erythromycin, trimethoprim-sulfamethoxazole, and quinolones.

- Penicillin is in the antibiotic group known as the beta-lactams, which bind to proteins on the bacterial cell wall surface and then interfere with a bacterial enzyme that is involved in creating the cross-linkages among the outer layer of the bacterial cell wall.

- In the 1940s, Englishman Howard Florey and German-born Ernst Chain learned how to extract penicillin and produce it in sufficient amounts to test in animals. Penicillin was subsequently released for human testing for those who were considered near death, often with dramatically favorable results. Florey also managed to convince the U.S. government to support large-scale production, and penicillin was made available in both intravenous and oral forms.

- Sulfonamides are another class of antibiotics. In the 1930s, Gerhard Domagk, a German professor, was examining an assortment of chemical dyes for their possible antibacterial effect. One manmade dye, called protonsil, was active against mice infected with streptococcal bacteria.

- Sulfonamides work by disrupting the pathway that leads to the synthesis of DNA. Folic acid is a building block needed for DNA synthesis that structurally resembles sulfonamides. The two compounds compete to acquire an enzyme known as para-aminobenzoic acid, which is necessary for folate production and subsequent DNA synthesis. Derivatives of the sulfonamide drugs over the next few decades formed one of the key foundations for antimicrobial therapy and continue to be used today.

- In 1943, streptomycin, the first drug useful for tuberculosis (TB) treatment, was discovered. The bacterium that produces streptomycin was found in a farmer's field. Not only was streptomycin able to treat TB, but it was also useful to cure gram-negative bacterial infections, which penicillin could not. However, when streptomycin was used alone for TB, resistance emerged. Also, damage by streptomycin to the kidneys prompted further development of an improved antibiotic, neomycin.

- Both drugs belong to the class of antibiotics known as aminoglycosides. They exert their mechanism of action by inhibiting protein synthesis. They bind to the ribosomes of bacteria, and this causes an inaccurate reading of messenger RNA, so proteins are synthesized erroneously. More advanced aminoglycoside derivatives are still in use today.

- So far, the antibiotics discovered attacked either gram-positive or gram-negative bacteria, but not both. In 1947, a Yale researcher discovered an antibiotic from a soil sample collected in a field in Caracas, Venezuela, and named it chloramphenicol. This was the first broad-spectrum antibiotic to exhibit activity against germs with different cell walls and different gram-staining characteristics.

- Chloramphenicol was found to interrupt protein synthesis by interfering with the binding of messenger RNA at ribosomes, similar to aminoglycosides. This antibiotic was a first-line drug for typhus and typhoid fever in the mid-1900s. Unfortunately, a rare idiosyncratic side effect of total blood-cell production shutdown occurred in a tiny percentage of treated patients, but this was enough to taint the use of chloramphenicol.

- In 1948, another broad-spectrum antibiotic named aureomycin was being studied. This was the prototype for the class of drugs we know today as tetracyclines. Its mechanism of antibacterial action is blocking the attachment of transfer RNA at the ribosome site of protein synthesis. With their broad spectrum of activity and rare side effects, tetracyclines emerged as a major class of antibiotic that we still use today—second only to beta-lactam penicillins.

- Erythromycin is another antibiotic class used for nearly 50 years, with a nearly identical mechanism of action to the tetracyclines.

- In the 1970s, trimethoprim was introduced as a synthetic antimicrobial. A novel idea occurred to chemists that if they combined two antibiotics at different steps in the same crucial folate metabolic pathway, the combined drugs would be more effective at interrupting DNA synthesis. This resulted in trimethoprim-sulfamethoxazole, which is still one of the first-line antibiotics chosen for the treatment of bladder infections and is also effective for MRSA.

- The final class of antibiotics is also synthetic drugs derived from a compound, nalidixic acid. This prototype was used for the development of the broad-spectrum class known as quinolone antibiotics, which were introduced in the 1980s.

- The mechanism of action of the quinolone drugs is unique, because they bind to a crucial enzyme called DNA gyrase, which is responsible for the unzipping of DNA during reproduction of bacteria. Due to widespread use as a broad-spectrum "kill everything" antibiotic, not surprisingly, resistance has emerged. Unfortunately, quinolones are also exploited for food and growth promotion in livestock animals, also leading to resistance that has sometimes been transferred to humans.

Antibiotic Use, Overuse, and Resistance

- For every mechanism of action of an antibiotic, we can virtually be assured that there is a mechanism of resistance. When bacteria divide, they duplicate their DNA, proteins, and cell walls. They also replicate at a rapid rate, and each time there is a division of cells, there is a chance for genetic mutations of any of these three cell products. The genetic mutation can occur at the level of the genes within chromosomes or in extra-chromosomal genes that exist in the cytoplasm of cells, known as plasmids.

- There are ample opportunities for bacteria to share genetic material, including many genes that can encode for resistance. The mechanisms of bacterial resistance can be divided into four general categories: enzyme inactivation; altered bacterial membrane target site; altered other target site, such as a ribosome; and antibiotic efflux pumps.

- In 2013, the CDC issued a summary report on the emerging crisis of antimicrobial resistance, including the names of the bacteria on the "watch list." The top three bacteria on the resistance "hot list" include *Clostridium difficile*, which causes serious diarrhea; *Neisseria gonorrhea*; and drug-resistant gram-negative bacteria that produce a beta-lactamase enzyme called CRE against our newest antibiotics. Other serious threats include resistant strains of MRSA, pneumococcus, salmonella, and tuberculosis.

- The development of new antibiotics has stalled over the past two decades. This includes the inability to discover new molecular targets in bacteria and the failure to find target drugs that exhibit antimicrobial properties.

- Another disturbing problem is that there are disincentives to the pharmaceutical industry to develop drugs that are only taken for a limited period of time, which have limited financial incentive when compared with drugs for chronic illness, such as hypertension or diabetes. Since 1983, there has been a stunning decline in the number of antibiotics discovered.

- But we can improve the use of our current antibiotics. In particular, this means not requesting antibiotics from your doctor when they

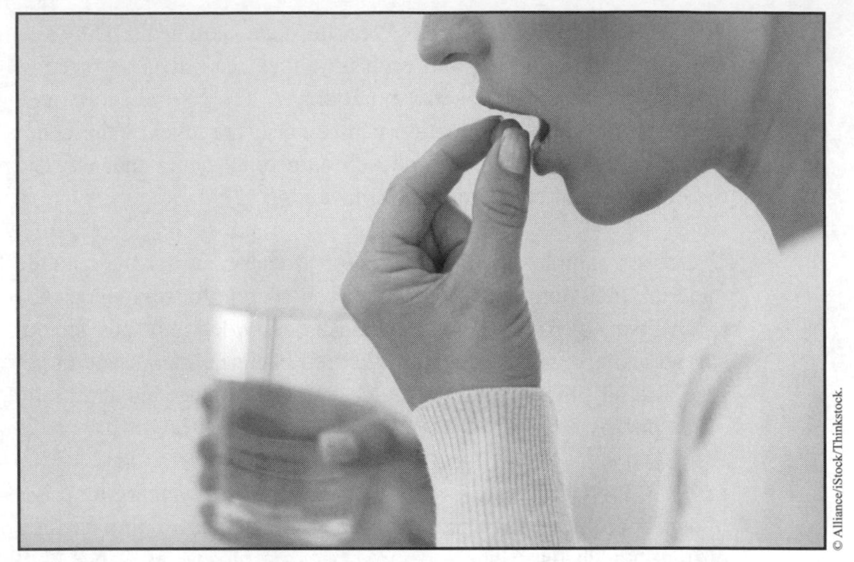

In the field of medicine, there is a tendency to overprescribe antibiotics, resulting in greater antibiotic immunity in the population.

determine that they are unnecessary and ineffective—especially in cases of viral illness. This is likely the most important action to slow the rate of drug-resistant microbes.

- Why is there a discrepancy between prescribing habits and the actual need? There are factors in motion that can easily lead to antibiotic overprescribing. From a patient standpoint, a patient might have been treated with antibiotics in the past for the same condition and had the impression, correctly or not, that he or she improved due to the antibiotic. From a health-care provider perspective, it takes time to explain to a patient why he or she might not need an antibiotic.

- Health-care providers also want to satisfy their patients' expectations, due to the concern that the same patient might go down the street to another provider that prescribes antibiotics. The situation is only magnified by the acuity of illness, meaning that visits to urgent care centers and emergency departments are likely to have even more implicit pressure to yield an antibiotic prescription.

- The Centers for Disease Control and Prevention has been aware of this patient-provider paradox for at least the past decade and initiated a campaign known as Get Smart to educate patients and families about the need, risk, benefits, and side effects associated with antibiotic prescriptions. It also provides educational tools for health-care providers to make it easier for patients to understand why antibiotics might not be appropriate.

- The use of antibiotics kills not only the intended bacteria, but also has collateral damage on the good bacteria. This has made *Clostridium difficile* the top urgent health-care threat to the United States, because this illness is caused by overgrowth of bad bacteria in the colon. From our society's perspective, we all have a vested interest in ensuring that antibiotics are prescribed only when necessary.

- Patients in the hospital have little or no choice in the decision-making process of whether they receive antibiotics there or not. Over the past decade, a concept has evolved known as antimicrobial stewardship, the goal of which to use antibiotics wisely and safely. A stewardship team is composed of pharmacists, infectious disease physicians, and microbiologists who review antibiotic-prescribing habits in the hospital for each individual patient as well as overall antibiotic-prescribing trends.

- Another dimension in antimicrobial resistance is the widespread use of antibiotics in food-producing animals, which amazingly accounts for nearly 80 percent of antibiotic use overall. More than 75 percent of this use is for fattening the animals. This use, especially with subtherapeutic antibiotic concentrations, contributes to the emergence of antibiotic-resistant bacteria in food-producing animals that can be transmitted to humans.

- Fortunately, there are legislative efforts moving forward in the United States that bring pharmaceutical manufacturers, the American Dairy Association, and health departments together to agree to limit the use of antibiotics in food-producing animals to medicinal purposes only.

- To stimulate new antibiotic development, the FDA is also trying to motivate pharmaceutical companies to devote time and money to the research and development of new antibiotics, including passing the Generating Antibiotic Incentives Now Act. The FDA can also designate a potentially new antibiotic for "fast track" status and priority FDA review.

- In 2014, President Obama also issued both an executive order and a U.S. national strategy to combat antibiotic resistant bacteria, which included establishing a task force for combating resistant bacteria, requiring all federal health programs to have antimicrobial stewardship, strengthening national surveillance and international collaboration efforts against resistant bacteria, and promoting the development of next-generation antibiotics.

Suggested Reading

Hager, Thomas, *The Demon under the Microscope*.

Lax, *The Mold in Dr. Florey's Coat*.

Levy, *The Antibiotic Paradox*.

Sachs, *Good Germs, Bad Germs*.

Questions to Consider

1. Can you imagine what it was like trying to treat infectious diseases without antibiotics? What treatments would we currently be using?

2. Why are we in danger of losing the "miracle" of these modern drugs? What do you think the future of antibiotics is?

Which Germs in Your Daily Life Matter?
Lecture 7

We are all exposed to a huge variety of germs every day. In this lecture, you will learn some hints for how you can protect yourself from germs without becoming totally obsessed about them. Just because there are germs on a door handle or a pepper shaker does not mean that you will automatically become ill by using or touching these objects. However, the goal of this lecture is to make you cognizant of specific circumstances where pathogenic viruses or bacteria may be avoided—with a little knowledge from this lecture and some common sense.

Germs in the Home

- There are at least several billion microorganisms keeping you company in your own home. Most of them are harmless, but some could be potentially dangerous. The kitchen is one of the dirtiest places in the home. The kitchen floor just in front of the sink has more bacteria than the trash can, and the sponges around the sink own a large burden of bacteria. You can sterilize a wet sponge by putting it in the microwave for two minutes.

- If you wash chicken in the kitchen sink and either a sponge falls in the sink or you turn on the faucet with unwashed hands, both the sponge and the faucet can become contaminated with virulent intestinal pathogens, such as campylobacter or salmonella.

- When you flush a toilet, bacteria in the toilet disperse in the air, and anything within a three-foot radius could be contaminated. So, close the lid if you can. Even toothbrushes lying around can be contaminated. In fact, the average toothbrush after brushing has about 10 million germs. However, as long as you use your own toothbrush, these are your bacteria and are not harmful.

- Sharing toothbrushes could pass on blood-borne viral diseases, such as hepatitis B and C, and infectious mononucleosis. Other things to watch out for are sharing makeup, which may result in sharing bacteria, and sharing razors, which may also inadvertently share MRSA or blood-borne viruses.

- Leave your shoes at the door. You not only keep the house cleaner, but you also don't track in allergens and potential pathogenic germs. One study found that as many as nine different pathogenic bacteria were in the dirt and other assorted things stuck to shoes. You can then transmit them to tile or carpeting all over your home.

- In terms of personal electronic devices, if you are the only one using your tablet, laptop, or cell phone, you're likely OK, because the germs are your own. However, be careful where you place these devices. Studies have shown that 16 percent of cell phones have intestinal bacteria on them.

- In general, cold and flu germs from sneezes can live on hard surfaces for up to 48 hours. The swine flu has been shown to survive in the environment for up to five days. Think about this before you hand your cell phone over to your sick spouse, family member, or friend.

- Germs on technology devices and elsewhere have opened up new markets of products to kill germs and protect you in the process. It's difficult to clean your tablet or laptop with bleach or alcohol, but new products are emerging, such as washable screen protectors and disposable covers that enclose the entire device. These may be particularly useful in health-care environments, where there is a huge potential for pathogens to easily get from hands to tablets or computers.

- One research project found thousands of bacteria on the Amtrak touch screen in a train station. If you use touch screens—including ones in grocery stores, ATMs, ticket kiosks, and airport check-ins—wash your hands thoroughly afterward. Washing your hands is the only thing that can significantly reduce your chances of getting sick.

Travel-Related Germs

- A study was done in 2011 on sites of possible contamination during a cross-country trip—for example, in a personal car, on commuter train seats, and in a taxi. The findings showed hundreds of bacteria on the rental car seats, as well as staphylococcus on train and taxi seats. Most of these are nonpathogenic bacteria. Even if there are some potential pathogens, such as *E. coli*, our immune systems should be strong enough to prevent major illness.

- Every pole you hold onto on the train, bus, or subway has the possibility of spreading cold-and-flu viruses and bacteria. Viruses are more likely to cause illness than bacteria, because the mucous membranes of the nose and eyes are more easily breached by viruses.

- There has been speculation that contaminated air circulating in an airplane is responsible for spreading germs. However, a revealing study now cites low cabin humidity as the biggest culprit if you become ill. At low levels of humidity, around 10 percent when flying at 30,000 to 35,000 feet, the mucous membranes in our noses and throats become drier.

- In a normal environment, viruses and bacteria are trapped and moved on by the cilia, or hairlike sweepers, to be destroyed by infection-fighting white blood cells. When the membranes are dry, the mucus may become too thick to move easily; therefore, the viruses and bacteria stay in the upper respiratory tract for longer periods of time. This low-humidity factor also applies to wintertime conditions for transmission of germs.

- According to multiple sources, the worst place on the plane for germs is likely the restroom on the plane, but there are many areas that are a close second, including airplane trays or aisle-seat handles. Of course, with many people in small spaces, there are more opportunities to share germs directly from person to person.

- The most dangerous neighbors on a plane are those sitting within a two-seat radius. Importantly, six to eight feet constitutes a safe distance that bacteria and viruses cannot readily be transmitted by aerosolized means of coughing or sneezing, because most bacteria or viruses will fall to the ground in that distance. This makes it difficult to keep your distance from seated neighbors on a plane.

- Airplane air is as well protected as the inside of a hospital. Airplanes have high-efficiency air particulate filters, which filter more than 90 percent of known particulate matter, including those that may be suspended in the air. So, don't worry too much—just take appropriate precautions if you can for sneezing neighbors.

- In a recent study, in a restaurant, menus carried the most germs, followed by the pepper shaker. Most of these bacteria were harmless, but you can't control an unusual germ. Protect yourself as far as your common sense can take you, and then relax and eat.

- Concerns that the bedspread on hotel beds is an item that doesn't get cleaned often enough may be well founded. Some scientists have recommended removing this item. In addition, one study found that light switches and bathroom floors were all contaminated with intestinal bacteria, but the dirtiest site was the TV remote.

- Gyms are a haven for germs. You can contract illnesses by moving from machine to machine, touching handles, changing weights, and lying on mats—often sitting in other people's sweat. Most gyms now supply cleaning solutions and towels to wipe down the equipment, so use them. And keep any cuts or injuries fully covered when working out at the gym.

- Also, both plantar wart (a virus) and athlete's foot (a fungus) can be contracted by going barefoot on gym floors and locker rooms. So, wear shower shoes in the shower and locker room. If you're doing yoga, bring your own mat and wear socks until you get to it. This is especially important for "hot" yoga classes, where people sweat a lot.

How to Keep Yourself Well

- Many diseases are spread by coughing and sneezing. When you cough or sneeze, germs can travel up to six to eight feet. Using a tissue, or your hand, or a bent arm to cover your mouth and nose when coughing or sneezing can help stop the spread. Throw used tissues away, and clean your hands right afterward.

- On average, we touch our faces with our hands around 20 times per hour. So, try not to touch your eyes, nose, and mouth, which are the mucous membranes and provide easy access to your body for germs. Even when your hands appear to be clean, germs are often spread this way.

- Ultraviolet (UV) lights or wands utilize short-wavelength UV radiation that is harmful to microorganisms. These items are effective in destroying the nucleic acids in these organisms so that their DNA is disrupted by the UV radiation, leaving them unable to perform vital cellular functions. UV disinfection has a real role in hospital environments and has been used primarily in medical sanitation and increasingly has been employed to sterilize drinking water.

- Alcohol-based hand sanitizers contain 60 to 70 percent alcohol, so they can kill most germs instantly by denaturing, or twisting out of shape, proteins in bacteria and most viruses. Because they are convenient and can act quickly, within 15 seconds, they are widely used in hospitals and marketed in many stores. Note that alcohol is not selective: It kills both pathogenic bacteria as well as commensal, friendly bacterial flora.

- Research has shown that alcohol hand sanitizers do not necessarily pose any risk by eliminating "good" microorganisms that are naturally present on the skin. This is because your body quickly replenishes the good microbes on your hands. However, alcohol also strips the skin of the outer layer of oil, which may have negative effects on the barrier function of the skin.

- Germs can be transmitted unintentionally by unwashed hands. While alcohol hand gels work against many viruses, they unfortunately do not work very well with the norovirus, which is the most common cause of gastrointestinal illness in the United States.

- If you are using soap and water, you should wash your hands for about 24 seconds (two rounds of the "Happy Birthday" song), lathering fully and covering all sides of your fingers and hands to completely remove bacteria. If you wash your hands correctly with plain soap and water, you have a good chance of avoiding many opportunities to get sick.

- There are several kinds of antibacterial soaps. The most common contains a product called triclosan, which has been used for years in the health-care setting as a disinfectant. However, some animal research showed that it might disrupt our endocrine, or hormone, system.

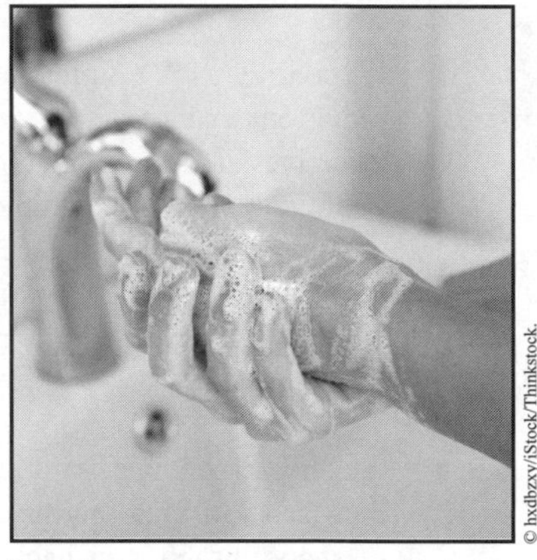

Washing your hands thoroughly and often can help you avoid getting sick.

- Besides soaps and gels, bleach is still known to be 99 percent effective as a disinfectant against pathogens, thanks to its active ingredient, hypochlorous acid. It attacks proteins in bacteria, causing them to clump together and die.

- A list of disinfectants that are registered with the Environmental Protection Agency can be found on its website. This list includes thymol, a derivative from the herb thyme. This can now be found even in bathroom cleaners made by companies that are responding to consumers' requests for less-toxic cleaning products.

- Another earth-friendly product, vinegar, is useful for killing some things but not others. For example, it is effective for killing the flu virus but not staph. It seems to be about 90 percent effective against bacteria and 80 percent against viruses. It is cheap, nontoxic, and biodegradable, and it has antimicrobial properties due to containing 5 percent acetic acid.

- The Internet is a good source for up-to-date green cleaner recipes. Tea tree oil may be added to commercial products, such as body wash, skin cream, and nasal ointment, due to its antimicrobial properties. Its structure appears to disrupt the cell membrane of MRSA.

- The "five-second rule" states that if you drop a piece of food, it is still OK to eat it if you pick it up within five seconds. Under most circumstances, this is probably OK. A 2014 study from England showed that time is a significant factor in the transfer of bacteria from a floor surface to a piece of food, and the type of flooring the food has been dropped on has an effect, with bacteria least likely to transfer from carpeted surfaces and most likely to transfer from laminate or tiled surfaces.

- Most germs that are crawling around our environment are usually commensal organisms and benign to most of us, but individuals with compromised immune systems, such as those receiving chemotherapy or taking moderate doses of steroid medications, should resist the urge to eat food that has been dropped on the ground or floor. And not every surface germ may be harmless.

Suggested Reading

Grossman, *Infection Control in the Child Care Center and Preschool.*

Rotbart, *Germ Proof Your Kids.*

Questions to Consider

1. Do you think it's realistic for you to take the time to sing the "Happy Birthday" song twice while washing your hands? If not, what is the alternative?

2. What are the germiest places in your own home? How can you take action to reduce the risk of contracting illnesses?

Six Decades of Infectious Disease Challenges
Lecture 8

This lecture examines infectious diseases decade by decade, from the prim-and-proper 1950s and radical 1960s to the present. In the 1950s, aside from poliomyelitis, it seemed like only a few other infectious diseases were nuisances to the American public: strep tonsillitis, childhood ear infections, and the common cold. Some scientists believed that the worst was over. But, in terms of infectious diseases, we have been on a roller coaster since the 1950s. And there will be more harrowing moments as new diseases, and possibly worldwide epidemics, emerge on the horizon.

Infections of the 1950s

- In children, the most common cause of tonsillitis is Group A streptococcus. Because it's a bacterium, strep will respond to antibiotics. But almost all tonsillitis will actually get better on its own. Antibiotics do shorten the duration of sore throat symptoms, but only by about 24 hours.

- The main reason we use antibiotics for streptococcal tonsillitis is because if left untreated, there is a small chance of developing rheumatic fever, which is an autoimmune disorder in which the body attacks itself. This is more serious than tonsillitis. Rheumatic fever was a leading cause of heart problems in the United States and is still the leading cause of heart disease in children from developing countries.

- It usually takes one to six weeks after the strep infection, if this rare autoimmune event is going to occur. Symptoms include fever, aching joints, sometimes a rash, and, if the heart is involved, symptoms of heart failure, such as sluggishness and fluid in the lungs.

- Rheumatic heart disease is still a common cause for the need for an artificial heart valve. Over the last several decades, the incidence of rheumatic fever has dramatically fallen in the United States, to less than one case per 100,000 people. So, in adults, the risk of developing rheumatic fever after strep pharyngitis is significantly less now, estimated at one chance in 5,000.

- Another circumstance that has dramatically changed over the past 50 years is the frequency of tonsillectomy surgeries in children for recurrent sore throats. In older days, most children had their tonsils removed, but now it's fairly unusual, unless there are consistent problems. However, there are still more than half a million tonsillectomies in the United States each year.

- Only 5 percent of pharyngitis in adults is due to Group A streptococcus; more than 90 percent are due to viral illnesses. That means that adults will rarely need antibiotics and are usually not at risk of developing rheumatic fever. How does a doctor know if it's just a sore throat or something more? The rapid office tests for Group A strep are very reliable.

- Another common illness of the mid-20th century from Group A strep was scarlet fever. Several days after a sore throat, children broke out with a lacy, almost-imperceptible rash on their entire body. In the 1950s, with penicillin available, children were usually kept home from school for a few days. In contrast, before the antibiotic era, this disease had almost a 25 percent mortality.

- These days, a 24-hour stretch of penicillin or similar antibiotics is considered enough time to render a child non-contagious to others. This is due to the rapid bacterial killing by penicillin, so the number of surviving germs is so low in 24 hours as to be considered non-contagious.

- Childhood ear infections are almost uniformly initially the result of a viral illness, and antibiotics are usually unnecessary. Children under age two are more prone to secondary, late bacterial ear infections. You should have children under two checked out by their doctor, provide pain relief for symptoms, and administer antibiotics only if the doctor thinks they are necessary.

- Onc of the most annoying illnesses is the common cold. Colds are caused by rhinoviruses and pester us for about a week. You are most contagious during the second and third days, when the viral burden is highest and coughing, sneezing, and congestion are at their peak. In adults, symptomatic over-the-counter cold medications can improve symptoms, although they are not recommended for small children.

- Around the world, there are various remedies for basic illnesses like a cold or the flu: In Israel, it's mint tea; in Russia, it's a drink called Gogol Mogol, which is made of raw egg, honey, warm milk, and butter, topped off with a shot of rum or cognac; and in Japan, it's a sour pickled plum called umeboshi. Most of these remedies have not been scientifically researched thoroughly, but they probably can't hurt and possibly might help. The best recommendation is to get extra rest, stay hydrated, and treat the symptoms of the illness.

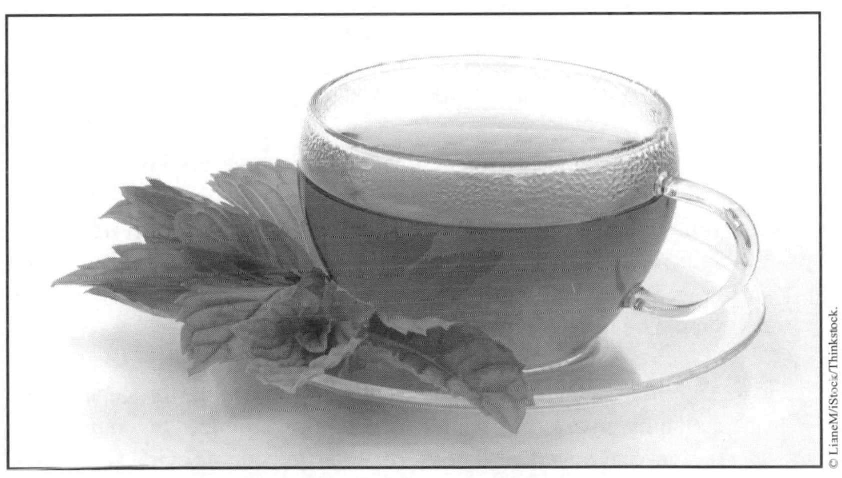

Although its effects have not been scientifically proven, mint tea is sometimes used as a remedy for a cold or the flu.

- Why, after all these years, don't we have a cure for the common cold? One huge problem is that there are more than 100 known cold viruses, so it's difficult to make a drug that could target all of them.

The 1960s

- While the 1950s was a decade of belief in science and its ability to conquer disease, the 1960s was a whole different era and would shake our confidence. The hippie generation of the 1960s brought some special infectious disease challenges, particularly related to risky behaviors.

- Sexual relations with multiple partners set the stage for a boom in sexually transmitted diseases (STDs). Intravenous drug experimentation led to the sharing of needles and the rise of hepatitis, meaning inflammation of the liver. Tattoos created with incompletely sterilized needles were another way that blood-sharing behaviors resulted in hepatitis.

- There is an alphabet soup of hepatitis viruses. Hepatitis A is usually connected with contaminated food and drinks and is spread by the fecal-oral route but does not cause permanent liver damage. Hepatitis B is transmitted through contaminated blood and sometimes through sexual conduct. Hepatitis C is usually acquired via contaminated blood and rarely sexual conduct.

- Worldwide, thousands of deaths are currently caused by hepatitis B and C, from eventual liver failure from decades of chronic infection. Today, hepatitis C is estimated to affect up to 3 million Americans, and the recommendation by the Centers for Disease Control and Prevention (CDC) is that all adults from the baby-boom generation should be tested.

- Antiviral medications were trialed in the 1990s for hepatitis C, including interferon, which is naturally produced by humans in response to any viral illness, so it has general antiviral properties. Eventually, interferon was commercially produced by recombinant DNA technology and became available for hepatitis treatment. Disappointingly, the clinical success rate of interferon for hepatitis C, even when combined with another antiviral medication called ribavirin, was no better than 50 percent remission.

- Other breakthroughs in treatment occurred after 2010 with the development of a protease inhibitor class of drugs that blocked the virus as it tried to exit liver cells. These protease inhibitors, when taken for 12 to 24 weeks, now give hepatitis C victims a chance to live virus-free.

The 1970s and 1980s

- In the 1970s, the outlook for handling emerging infectious diseases, even those that could start epidemics, appeared good. The United States was optimistic that it could handle whatever infectious diseases arose. There were improved sanitation, increased vaccination programs, and enough antibiotics that infectious diseases were on the decline. The financing for eradication of infectious diseases was now being diverted to other pressing diseases, such as chronic heart disease and cancer.

- However, the tide was about to dramatically change again. The end of the 1970s brought Legionnaires' disease, and the early 1980s brought the recognition of genital herpes and the slow discovery of human immunodeficiency virus (HIV). These three diseases urgently created a flurry of scientific activity to stem the tide of contagion and death.

- It took a while before health-care providers began sharing stories of a strange new illness in gay men in 1981. The CDC reported in its weekly journal a summary on five cases in previously healthy, young gay men with unusual infections, with immune systems that were dysfunctional. Within the next six months, 270 cases had been reported, with 121 deaths. The AIDS epidemic was born.

- The discovery of HIV as the cause for AIDS, and the subsequent blood test that was developed for HIV in 1985, were major achievements in medicine in a short time. However, infectious disease doctors had to care for patients with AIDS without any medications to treat the root cause, the HIV virus. If the patient had a bacterial infection, doctors could provide them with hope by using antibiotics to at least cure their bacterial infections.

- HIV rose to celebrity status when Rock Hudson died of the disease in 1985, and by then, he had donated money to set up the American Foundation for AIDS Research, chaired by Elizabeth Taylor. More than 36 million people have died of AIDS-related illnesses, and it is the most common cause of infectious disease death in the world by a single illness.

- There was somewhat of a reversal in public attitude toward AIDS as it spread throughout the world. We were facing a worldwide epidemic of AIDS, along with several other concerning infectious diseases. This was just the beginning of new, emerging infectious diseases that would plague the world for decades to come.

The 1990s

- The 1990s brought some new medical developments, such as chicken pox vaccines, as well as novel antiviral drugs to treat both hepatitis and HIV. But we were also learning more about a viral illness that has infected nearly all of us: the Epstein-Barr virus (EBV).

- This virus got its name in 1964 when Sir Michael Epstein and Yvonne Barr discovered it. A few years later, the virus was linked to infectious mononucleosis, which is usually transmitted via saliva. Symptoms include generalized fatigue lasting for more than a few weeks, a persistent sore throat that tests negative for strep, fevers, enlarged lymph nodes, and possibly an enlarged spleen.

- The major discovery in the 1990s about EBV was something that is true for all herpes viruses: the ability to establish a dormant, or latent, infection—somewhat like chicken pox coming back as shingles. EBV was also found to have the ability to cause cancer.

The New Millennium

- When we crossed the millennium, another major achievement of modern medicine was accomplished: We were able to give premature babies as young as 28 weeks old a chance at survival. These premature infants had virtually no immune system of their own, which made them vulnerable to many infectious germs, but especially to a virus known as respiratory syncytial virus (RSV). RSV is an RNA virus that is known to cause giant conglomerations of virus particles.

- More importantly, the lungs of these premature newborns had such immature airways that the children were vulnerable to RSV attacking the lungs, closing off the airways, and leading to death—without any treatment available. Eventually, an antiviral medication, ribavirin, was used for treatment if an infection developed, and immune serum was given weekly for prevention. This saved many infants' lives.

- As we turn the page of the millennium further, we are forced to confront a viral nemesis that remains of epidemic magnitude: norovirus infections. This is an illness that all age groups are susceptible to, because it's food-borne.

- Noroviruses are the most common food-borne disease in the United States and the most frequent cause of intestinal illness. They produce nausea and vomiting and often rapid-onset diarrhea. Fever is common for 24 hours. The illness usually lasts for a maximum of 48 to 72 hours with a rapid and full recovery but, unfortunately, without long-lasting immunity.

- Norovirus causes an estimated 1 in 15 U.S. residents to become ill each year. Deaths can occur among young children and the elderly, due to severe dehydration. Food handlers cause 70 percent of norovirus outbreaks by contaminating food and by touching fruit, vegetables, or bread with ungloved hands.

- Norovirus is extremely contagious, because it can survive on surfaces for days. You need to wash your hands with soap and water and not rely on alcohol gels. It can also survive freezing and cooking temperatures above 140 degrees.

- Within the past year, one in five restaurant workers admits having reported to work while sick with vomiting or diarrhea. This has led to a CDC recommendation that paid sick leave be offered as an incentive to stay home and be symptom-free for 48 hours before returning to work.

Suggested Reading

Henderson, *Smallpox*.

Questions to Consider

1. Which challenges regarding infectious diseases do you think will define the first two decades of the 21st century?

2. Which diseases do you think will be eradicated, or have a cure or vaccine, by 2025?

Vaccines Save Lives

Lecture 9

The subject of this lecture is vaccinations and immunizations. In this lecture, you will learn the importance of vaccines and their ability to prevent a devastating illness and even death. You will learn about the development of vaccines, the types of vaccines, and the substantial impact that vaccines have on health in the United States and abroad. There is a definitive cause-and-effect relationship between vaccination and its effect on the emergence of disease in individuals and in populations.

Vaccine Development

- Edward Jenner, at the turn of the 19th century, ingeniously created a smallpox vaccine that used cowpox, a cousin of smallpox, to protect against the disease but not cause serious illness. There was skepticism in early America about the efficacy of the vaccine, so the Board of Health of Boston, founded in 1779 and chaired by Paul Revere, formulated a clinical trial of the vaccine to prove or disprove its effectiveness—the first controlled human trial that convinced the public that the vaccine worked and was safe.

- The smallpox vaccine is no longer a cowpox derivative. Instead, in the late 19th century, a new live vaccine derived from a similar virus, the vaccinia virus, replaced cowpox. It starts giving protection against smallpox a few days after it is given. It provides immunity for at least three to five years, and longer if booster shots are given. This relatively quick immune response would be important for rapid protection in response to smallpox bioterrorism.

- Vaccine development traditionally has been a long, complex process, sometimes lasting a decade or more and involving a combination of public and private resources. Vaccines are developed, tested, and regulated in a manner very similar to antibiotics. This includes oversight by the Food and Drug Administration (FDA) in collaboration with the CDC's Immunization Safety Office.

- The exploratory stage usually lasts two to four years and consists of basic lab research. Scientists identify natural or synthetic antigen proteins as targets. Preclinical activities involve using cultures and animal testing to assess safety. Many vaccines never get beyond this point. If they do, a sponsor submits an application for an investigational new drug to the FDA.

- If approved, it goes through three stages of rigorous testing, including clinical studies with human subjects in small groups, and then in larger and larger groups. Safety is tested as well as efficacy. If successful, it usually is approved.

- In order to encourage vaccine development in the United States, the government removed liability responsibility from pharmaceutical developers for approved vaccines. The United States has a national vaccine injury compensation program for anyone injured by a vaccine.

- In order to mass-produce vaccines, viruses and bacteria have to be grown in large quantities. They also have to be meticulously produced to ensure consistent results. Bacteria can be grown in a liquid growth medium, where they rapidly multiply. Viruses are more difficult to grow, because they have to use living cells. Viruses are grown in immature, or embryonic, eggs or tissues or in primitive cell line cultures.

- Another boost for the vaccine movement occurred in 1941, when the rubella virus was found to cause fetal abnormalities in pregnant women. Fetuses with mothers infected with rubella had congenital heart conditions, deafness, and mental retardation. This conveyed an urgent need to develop a rubella vaccine.

- Four groups of scientists managed to attenuate, or weaken, the live rubella virus—three from primary animal cells and one from human cells. The rubella vaccine was the first vaccine created with the use of human cell lines.

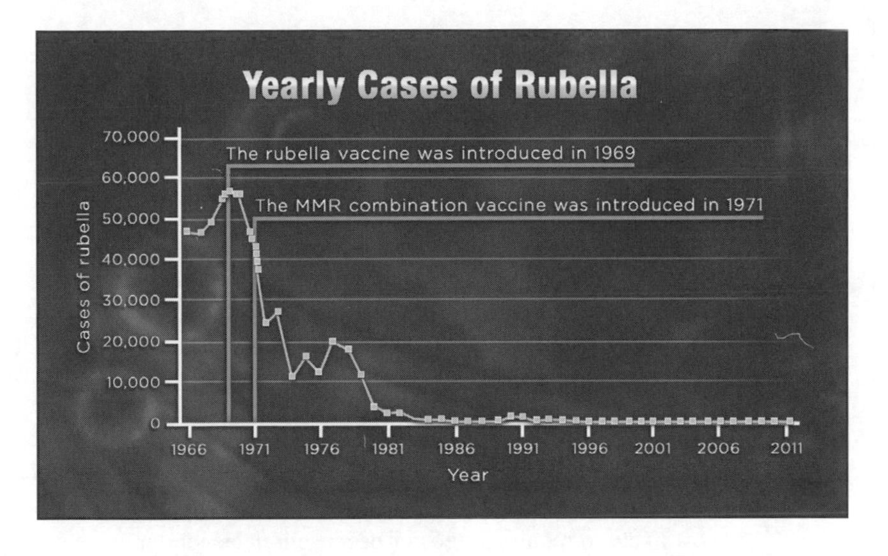

- Virologist Stanley Plotkin grew the virus through cell lines 25 times at a lower-than-normal body temperature of 86 degrees in order to weaken the virus so that it would no longer be infectious. Rather, it was just strong enough to provoke an immune response.

- Interestingly, the three animal cell vaccines were approved in 1969 and 1970 in the United States, and the human vaccine was only approved in Europe. Evidently, there was bias against using human cells for fear of contamination. Eventually, the human vaccine not only replaced the animal cell line vaccines, but Plotkin's vaccine is still used in the measles-mumps-rubella vaccine given to children today.

Types of Vaccines

- Vaccines can be made in several different ways.
  - Using live viruses that are weak enough not to cause disease.
  - Using inactivated (killed) bacteria or viruses.
  - Using inactivated toxins, known as toxoids, of bacterial germs.
  - Using a portion of the germ coating.

- We need to use four different types of vaccines because different microorganisms have more ideal targets to maximize our body's immune response. For example, although we have been working on an HIV vaccine for more than a decade, the ideal target for vaccination has yet to be identified.

- How do we decide which type of vaccine to use for which disease? The live, attenuated vaccine, as described for the rubella virus, is too weak to cause significant illness but strong enough to provoke an immune response that protects against future infection.

- Inactivated, or killed, vaccines are made by inactivating a pathogen, typically using heat or chemicals, such as formaldehyde. This destroys the pathogen's ability to replicate, but keeps it intact so that the immune system can still recognize it. This type of vaccine is most likely to require a booster because it does not duplicate the normal infection process in humans.

- Toxoids are different because the diseases they cause are not from the bacterium itself, but from a toxin produced by the bacterium. Immunizations can be made by inactivating the toxin using chemicals or heat.

- Both subunit and conjugate vaccines contain only pieces of the pathogens they protect against. Conjugate vaccines, however, are made using pieces from the outer coatings of bacteria that are then chemically linked to a carrier protein, and the combination is used as a vaccine. The carrier protein is often chosen to maximize the human immune response to the entire complex—not just the bacterial coating. Essentially, we are tricking our own immune system into a maximum response.

- The first vaccines available for influenza were killed, but there has been progress with both live vaccines and so-called high-dose killed vaccines. The high-dose influenza vaccine is now the vaccine of choice for adults over the age 65.

- In general, live vaccines mimic the actual infectious process better than inactivated vaccines and thereby result in a stronger and longer immune response. Hence, it has been recommended that children ages 2 to 8 get the live influenza vaccines. They may even transfer the live vaccine to others, enhancing a concept known as herd immunity, which describes the number of people in a community that must be vaccinated in order for the entire community to be protected. Typically, this is between 80 and 95 percent, depending on the particular disease. This is the herd immunity threshold.

- But this also means that 5 to 20 percent of the population, if not vaccinated, are essentially freeloaders on the rest of society. If the high threshold is maintained, the non-vaccinated may not get ill. But if the threshold falls too low, the non-vaccinated may contract the illness and spread it to others.

The Anti-Vaccination Movement

- Even back in the mid-1800s, vaccines were deemed compulsory in Britain. There were severe punishments for not being vaccinated, including fines and imprisonment, because they recognized that everyone's health was interconnected. Some people said that this was a violation of civil liberty. Fifty years later, the law was amended to allow for conscientious objections.

- There has been much chatter in the press about the recent anti-vaccination movement. Some anti-vaccinationists say that they had chickenpox, measles, and mumps as a child and got through it just fine. We know that natural infections can have a negative influence on childhood development and can cause complications or even death.

- Some anti-vaccinationists say that they are afraid that vaccines will cause autism or other disorders because they contain mercury. Coincidentally, autism emerged around the timing of the current vaccination schedule for a one-year-old child, so the occurrence can be misleading. Numerous vaccines are given to babies over the first year just when many developmental changes occur. If something happens around this time, often the vaccine is blamed.

- Certain vaccines contain ingredients like formaldehyde, aluminum, phenol, or mercury, but only in minute concentrations and always below a healthy threshold. Formaldehyde's purpose is to kill the vaccine's viruses, ensuring its safety. Aluminum hydroxide enhances the immune response, and phenol acts as a preservative, which is especially important when vaccines are being sent overseas and need to maintain their stability for a period of time.

- Thimerosal is a mercury-containing ingredient that was used in many vaccines to prevent the growth of bacteria. It is no longer used in the United States in any routine childhood vaccines. In fact, though, no scientific studies have found a connection between autism and thimerosal in vaccines.

- Another concern for some individuals is that for vaccines made with live viruses, there's a chance that you can acquire the disease that the viral vaccination was meant to protect. It's true that certain vaccines can cause mild symptoms of the disease itself. One example is varicella/chicken pox, which contains an attenuated form of the live virus. Mild pox rashes may occur in about five percent of vaccines.

- Some parents think that there are too many vaccines in the first six months; they are worried that the vaccines cause overloads on the babies' immune systems. The current recommended vaccine schedule can include up to 23 shots by the time children are 2 years old and as many as 6 shots at a single doctor's visit. So, it's not surprising that people are concerned. But doctors believe that children have an enormous capacity to respond safely to challenges to their immune system.

- Some anti-vaccinationists say that because vaccines are not 100 percent effective and also don't give lifelong protection, the risks of vaccination outweigh the benefits. Some vaccinations, such as chicken pox and hepatitis A, are thought to grant lifelong immunity. Other vaccinations may last only 5 to 10 years, and the flu shot only covers you for one year, because the influenza virus strains are different every year and a new vaccine must be developed.

- Part of the decision whether or not to get vaccinated depends on your individual response to illness—that is, how strong your immune system is. People who are elderly or chronically ill are particularly at risk for debilitating symptoms or even death from the flu.

- Depending on your age and health and the strain of flu virus that is circulating, it protects between 50 to 90 percent of those vaccinated. The vaccine is usually less effective at older ages and those with compromised immune systems, but the high-strength flu vaccine already has shown promise for improved protection. Also, flu vaccines now contain four strains of virus, not three.

The Future of Vaccinations

- Vaccination requirements are likely to continue to get tougher in the future. Influenza vaccination is already uniformly recommended for all children ages six months and older, and it is now being required for preschool and daycare in most states.

- Legislation has just passed the first stages of Congress that would require a physician's note for families declining vaccinations. It would need to state that the physician had counseled the parents regarding the consequences of non-vaccination. And the time has come, at least at most local levels, when many health-care institutions have made influenza vaccinations mandatory as a condition for providing health care to the general public.

- Should you be concerned about receiving vaccinations as an adult? Vaccination recommendations are usually in a state of flux. Make sure that you review your vaccine history with your health-care provider at any medical visit, not just a routine physical, especially the following items.

- A tetanus and diphtheria booster every 10 years. After age 50, at least one booster should contain the whooping cough component. You don't have to wait until age 65 for the tetanus-diphtheria-acelluar pertussis vaccine.

- If you haven't gotten the full vaccination series as a child, you should review that with your doctor, especially if you are regularly around babies or the elderly.

- If you are 60 or older, get information on the shingles vaccine, and if you are over 65, get information on the two choices of pneumonia vaccines.

- If traveling, make sure to check with your travel medicine clinic.

Suggested Reading

Cave, *What Your Doctor May Not Tell You about Children's Vaccinations*.

O'Shea, *Vaccination Is Not Immunization*.

Questions to Consider

1. Do you think vaccinations will replace antibiotics some day?

2. Do you think vaccinations should be required for all levels of education? What is your view on exemptions?

The Immune System: Our Great Protector

Lecture 10

Our immune systems are intricate collections of specialized cells, tissues, and molecules that work together to protect us from infectious diseases. When our immune system is working well, we stay healthy; when it's not, we may become susceptible to deadly infections or even develop an autoimmune disorder. In this lecture, you will learn about the components of the immune system and how they work together to protect us. In addition, you will learn what happens to the immune system as we age and what we can do to boost our immune system.

Components of the Immune System

- The four structural components of the immune system include the thymus, bone marrow, the spleen, and the lymphatic system.
  - The thymus is a specialized organ located in front of your heart and behind your breastbone. It is responsible for producing T lymphocyte white blood cells.
  - Three different types of cells are produced in the bone marrow: red blood cells, blood-clotting elements called platelets, and white blood cells. The marrow is in the center of the bones.
  - The spleen is located in the left side of the abdomen. It synthesizes proteins known as antibodies and also gets rid of antibody-coated bacteria and old blood cells.
  - The lymphatic system is part of our circulatory system and is made up of a network of small vessels that carry a clear fluid called lymph. It works in tandem with lymphoid organs, especially lymph nodes. Lymphocyte immune cells are passed through this system and converge in the lymph nodes throughout the body.

The Innate Immune System

- There are two divisions of the immune system that we use to fight infections: innate immunity and adaptive immunity. We have certain built-in, or innate, immune features that help protect us when under attack. First, there are physical barriers to invasion from microbes, including the skin and mucous membranes. These defenses do not target specific germs but are all-purpose defenses. Having intact skin and membranes helps prevent foreign invaders from entering the body. Other physical barriers include tears, mucus, saliva, and stomach acid.

- We have a few other lines of defense in our innate immunity. Our bodies have a common inflammatory response to invaders or injury. Damaged tissues release substances that start the inflammatory process.

- There are four cardinal signs of the inflammatory response. They have been written about since 3000 B.C. and still carry their Latin origins: rubor, or redness, which is caused by increased blood flow; dolor, or pain; calor, or warmth, which also is caused by increased blood flow; and tumor, or swelling caused by the movement of fluid into the area.

- There are types of white blood cells that help with the innate immune response. One type are neutrophils, which are one of the first lines of defense against foreign invaders and make up the largest number of white blood cells in your body. They are produced in the bone marrow and then become positioned along the margins of our circulatory system, and in the blood, acting as a reservoir of infection-fighting cells. What remains of neutrophils that are dead are what we know as pus.

- Another innate line of defense involves fever, raising body temperature, which means using the weapon of heat against a pathogen. There are many misperceptions of the benefits or dangers of fever. Fever impairs the ability of bacteria and viruses to replicate, creating an inhospitable environment for the invading organisms. By turning up the heat, invading microbes' metabolism and reproduction are skewed.

- The last component of the innate immune response is the complement system. This is a series of small protein molecules that help recruit inflammatory cells and enhance the destruction of germs. It works in tandem with neutrophils and proteins known as antibodies to engulf invaders.

The Adaptive Immune System

- The companion of innate immunity is the adaptive immune system. One difference between innate and adaptive immunity is that innate responses are nonspecific, meaning that they do not target specific pathogens. Another difference is that innate immunity has no memory of previous actions against pathogens. The two systems, though, work hand in hand.

- The adaptive immune system is composed of highly specialized cells that adapt to and learn from prior invaders. This is the system that remembers, for example, that you had measles as a child and will protect you for life against measles. The adaptive system has two major branches: the cell-mediated system and the antibody-mediated humoral system.

- Lymphocytes, another of the five types of white blood cells, carry out the immune responses in both branches of the adaptive system. Lymphocytes are divided into B cells and T cells. Fetal primitive stem cells that continue to mature in the bone marrow become B cells. Others complete their growth in the thymus and become T cells.

- Importantly, each B and T cell is specific for only one antigen, or foreign substance, so they can only bind to one particular molecular structure. B cells work in the humoral immune system and mount a very specific antigen response. B cells can also inactivate viruses by neutralizing them before they can enter host cells. Some B cells become memory cells, allowing a quicker and more specific immune response the next time the body encounters the same infection.

- T cells, on the other hand, are part of the cell-mediated immune response and can be divided further into helper T cells and cytotoxic T cells. In the case of HIV, the virus replicates quickly and destroys the helper T cells, resulting in more infected cells than healthy cells. Cytotoxic T cells attempt to destroy the HIV virus, but over time, the body's ability to fight off infection is severely depleted, making people with HIV highly susceptible to infections.

- T cells also activate B cells, and they can destroy microbes that are inside cells. Some T cells also transform into memory cells so that they will recognize their invader if it ever attacks again. Macrophages are present in essentially all tissues and are critical in both innate and adaptive immunity.

- Antibodies are the other major component of the humoral system. Antibodies are produced by B lymphocytes that have matured into plasma cells. They can perform several functions, including neutralizing bacterial toxins, binding to viruses to prevent entry into cells, and opsonization, in which a coating of antibodies increase the effectiveness of neutrophils trying to engulf bacteria. There are four main types of antibodies: immunoglobulins M, A, E, and G.

- It is imperative that there is communication and teamwork between the innate and adaptive immune systems to effectively fight off infections. Cytokines are chemical messengers that are secreted by various cells of the immune system to act on other cells and coordinate the immune responses.

- With an autoimmune condition, the immune system can't tell the difference between healthy body tissue and foreign antigens. The result is a T cell immune response that attacks normal body tissues, causing disorders such as lupus and multiple sclerosis. Some, but not most, autoimmune disorders have an infectious trigger, such as rheumatic fever.

The Immature Immune System of Newborns

- Much of a newborn's immune system is dependent on the transfer of immunity from the mother to the newborn before or during birth. The fetal immune system is derived from primitive stem cells, which arise from the inside of the bone structures of a developing fetus. These stem cells later differentiate into specialized cells as the immune system matures.

- It takes the newborn's immune system a minimum of four to six weeks to develop individual responsiveness. Because a child's initial vaccination series is not usually complete until age one and a half, those under one month of age, but also up to one year of age, are much more vulnerable to infections.

- Paradoxically, there are concerns, known as the hygiene hypothesis, that we are doing a potential disservice to the developing immune system by creating too clean of an environment. The developing immune system may need to be properly exposed to germs to function optimally. If the baby's environment is too clean, for example, the production of T-helper cells may not be adequately stimulated.

Aging and the Immune System

- While some people age in a healthy manner, the elderly are far more likely to contract infectious diseases. Respiratory infections, influenza, and particularly pneumonia are leading causes of death in those over age 65. No one knows for sure why this happens, but most scientists agree that this increased risk correlates with a decrease in T cells, possibly from the thymus shrinking with age and producing fewer T cells to fight off infection.

- The aging body also responds more slowly to challenges by infectious agents. Research has shown that with age, our innate defenses lose some of their ability for the cells to communicate with each other. If this happens, it makes it difficult for the cells to react timely and appropriately to invading germs.

- As a consequence of the reduction in production of lymphocytes, vaccination is not as likely to produce as strong of an immune response, both B cells and immunoglobulin. The response may even be below the threshold for protection.

- But despite the reduction in efficacy, vaccinations for influenza and pneumococcal pneumonia have significantly lowered the rates of sickness and death in older people when compared with non-vaccination. One exception to poor vaccine immune response appears to be good response to the shingles vaccine at age 60. Because one in three individuals over the age of 60 will develop shingles, it's important to get this vaccine.

- Because shingles is a reactivation of the chickenpox virus, it relies on our lymphocytes to remember prior viral exposure. Because we know this immune response will dwindle, if you have not gotten the vaccine, you need to be fastidious about recognizing the signs of shingles within 72 hours of symptoms. This is the window of opportunity for prescribing an antiviral drug for shingles. Medication may be effective in reducing both acute symptoms and the incidence of post-herpetic neuralgia.

- Be on the lookout for the following signs and symptoms.
    - Early twinging pains, itching, or unusual nerve sensitivity that is not attributable to injury.
    - Burning of the skin that is persistent in a limited area, followed by a red patch of skin without typical blisters.
    - For shingles of the head and eye, a sensation that there is something irritating your eye, but you can't find an eyelash or foreign object.

- One of the significant consequences of shingles, aside from the nuisance of the blisters and acute pain, is post-herpetic neuralgia, which occurs more frequently above age 60. This is intermittent or continuous pain of the nerves that were reactivated with infection.

Antiviral medication cannot alter the course of this pain if it's not given in the first 72 hours. Post-herpetic neuralgia can last for many months and make activities of daily living very difficult.

- Aside from the natural decline of the innate and active immune response, immune changes can also be the result of chemotherapy, radiation exposure, environmental exposures to toxins, and long-term stress.

- It's difficult to boost your immune system precisely because it is a system made up of many different types of cells. We're not sure exactly what kinds of cells and how many of them would make up a perfect system. The most prevalent advice by doctors on how to boost your immune system includes the following.
    - Eat a healthy diet.

    - Exercise.

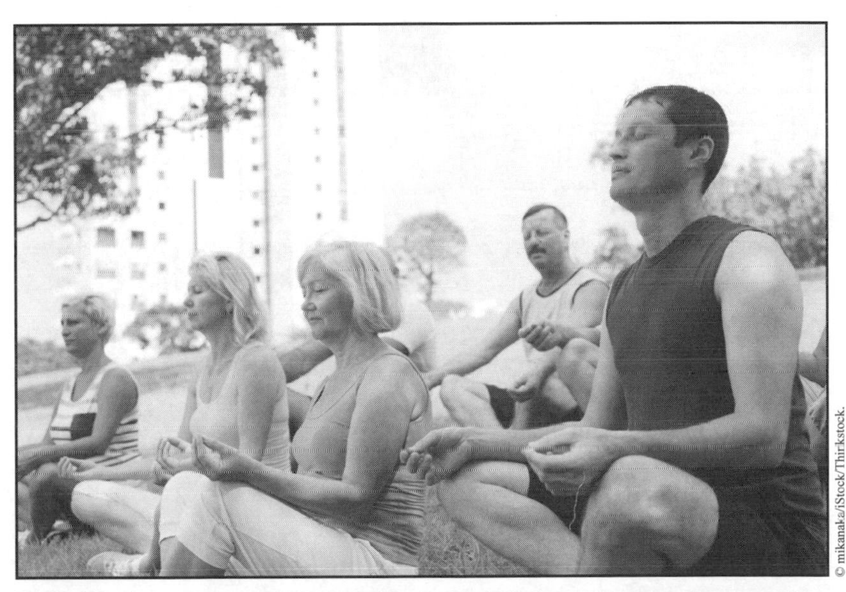

Meditation is a great way to reduce the amount of stress you experience, and stress reduction can boost your immune system.

- Avoid smoking.
- Control your blood pressure.
- Get your annual flu shot.
- Get your shingles vaccine at 60 and your pneumonia vaccine at 65.
- Reduce stress.

- One thing that has been added to the living healthy list is to practice meditation. Transcendental meditation has been recommended by the American Heart Association as a proven means to reduce blood pressure. Studies have shown that this method of meditation, practiced 20 minutes twice a day, also has had positive effects on reducing stress. Mindfulness meditation techniques may also be effective.

Suggested Reading

Abbas, Lichtman, and Pillai, *Basic Immunology*.

Sompayrac, *How the Immune System Works*.

Questions to Consider

1. Is fever helpful or hindering when there is an infectious condition? Would you take Tylenol for a fever of 100 degrees?

2. What is it about the immune system that makes us more susceptible to infection as we age? How does this affect how you will take care of yourself in the future?

Zoonosis: Germs Leap from Animals to Humans

Lecture 11

Today, diseases around the world are jumping from animals to humans at a faster pace than ever before. Why are new diseases so prevalent, and how are these exotic diseases being transmitted to people from animals? This phenomenon has been around for centuries, and more than 200 diseases have been identified as "zoonotic." In this lecture, you will learn about the reasons why transmission of diseases is occurring more frequently, the methods of transmission, the potential for human harm, and the prevention and containment of these diseases.

Rabies and Other Zoonotic Diseases

- Zoonosis is defined as any disease or infection that is naturally transmissible from animals with a backbone to humans. Infectious diseases aren't always spread just by exotic animals, but at times by our pets at home, including companion animals, and other common animals. Dogs and cats can also become the vectors of disease with contact with wild animals, potentially spreading germs to humans.

- The rabies virus has a bullet-like shape. After a bite, or even a scratch, by an infected animal, the virus can enter the body through the skin. If the wound goes unnoticed, which might occur with scratches, the virus establishes itself next in the local nerves where the injury occurred.

- Over the course of weeks or months, the virus is able to travel insidiously from the skin nerves to deeper nerves in the body. Immediate disinfection of the wound, and rabies immune-globulin injected into the wound site to confer passive immunity, are crucial urgent measures for protection.

- There is also a six-week rabies vaccination program that follows. Once local neurological symptoms develop, such as burning pain at the site and tingling of the nerves, the disease is almost uniformly fatal. As the virus spreads deeper into the body to the central nervous system, fatal inflammation of the brain and spinal cord develops. There are no reliable treatments available.

- Fortunately, in the United States, the strict adherence to rabies vaccination has made transmission of rabies from domestic animals to humans an extreme rarity. Nevertheless, today in several third-world countries, rabies might be transmitted from domestic animals, because they are often unvaccinated.

- In the United States, more than 90 percent of rabies comes from wildlife, especially bats. Other animals that harbor rabies include raccoons, skunks, and foxes. Around 40,000 people in the United States every year get rabies shots after exposure to wild animals. The estimated cost of receiving these vaccinations is more than $300 million dollars.

- Try to avoid the temptation to feed or handle wild animals. If you are bitten or scratched by a susceptible animal, wash the wound

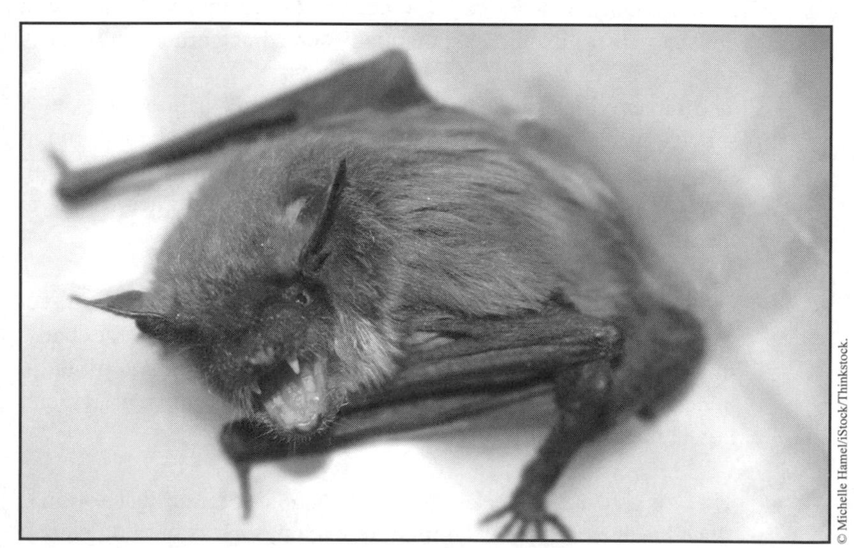

Wild animals, such as bats, are a major source of rabies.

with soap and water and get health-care attention quickly for post-exposure prevention. Try to have the domestic or wild animal captured by appropriately trained personnel. Then, notify the county animal health department so that the animal can either be sacrificed and tested for rabies or observed for rabies symptoms.

- Animals that might have rabies usually exhibit strange behavior patterns, especially a fear of water. If the animal is quarantined for 10 days without symptoms, additional rabies vaccinations can be avoided.

- Rabies is a preventable disease with the use of vaccines. For wild animals, one of the means of vaccination is by using oral rabies baits. This Wildlife Services program targets raccoons, coyotes, and foxes and is being used throughout the United States, Canada, and Europe.

- There are other zoonotic diseases related to dogs and cats that are also important. In the United States, there are more than 69 million dogs and 74 million cats, so it's important to consider infectious disease risks.

- One cat-transmittable disease is cat scratch disease, which is a bacterial disease caused by a germ known as *Bartonella henselae*. Most people with cat scratch illness have been bitten or scratched by a cat. They usually develop a mild infection near the injury site. Lymph nodes become swollen, and fever and flulike symptoms can occur for several days.

- Toxoplasmosis is another zoonosis transmitted by cats. Cats can become infected after eating infected tissue of rodents or, less commonly, cattle. Infectious cyst forms are shed by cats, and humans can become infected through accidental contact with feline fecal material. Surprisingly, most human infections, like cat infections, are asymptomatic. Other times, generalized whole-body lymph node enlargement, with flulike symptoms, can occur.

Small Pets Other Than Dogs and Cats

- Reptiles and amphibians, such as turtles, lizards, and frogs, can carry a harmful salmonella bacteria that causes intestinal illness. The salmonella infections can not only come from handling turtles, but also from the water or containers where they are living. Using gloves for cleaning the environments of the pets is essential, as is washing one's hands after handling them.

- Birds, baby chicks, and ducks are also sources of infectious diseases, including salmonella. In fact, chickens in certain environments, such as urban farms, can contract a parasite known as coccidia, which can be spread through chicken excrement, especially around feeders. This can be transmitted to humans and can cause diarrhea. One of the growing problems with urban farms is that regular veterinarians are not usually experienced with chickens and don't know how to properly diagnose or treat them.

- The Centers for Disease Control and Prevention has issued an alert that the surge in small urban farms is providing the perfect environment for an outbreak of salmonella. As people bring the chickens into their homes, they are letting them walk on tables and countertops and contaminating the home environment.

- Choose your pets wisely. Consider the age, environment, and health of all the people who might be in contact with the pets. The best thing you can do is educate yourself and children about potential health hazards of owning pets and implement stringent hand-washing practices.

- Other diseases may be transmitted from petting zoos, regular zoos, or farms. Petting zoo animals can shed a variety of germs without the animals appearing ill. Most concerning are young children, who may touch an animal and then put their hands in their mouths or on food. There have been numerous outbreaks of disease at petting zoos, including bacterial and parasitic germs that usually cause intestinal symptoms that include vomiting and/or diarrhea.

- Another potential cause for alarm for cute and furry pets relates to pet stores and rodents. Pet rodents, such as hamsters and guinea pigs, can asymptomatically carry a virus called lymphocytic choriomeningitis virus, which can cause inflammation around the brain and spinal cord. Fortunately, human infections from pet rodents are rare.

Wildlife Animals

- Hantavirus is a rare but serious disease that humans can contract through contact with infected urine, saliva, or droppings from rodents. Dried urine in dust carries virus particles, and sweeping the dust or pitching a tent in an infected area can cause inhalation of the virus. This can lead to a life-threatening bleeding disorder of the lungs, with no available treatment.

- Whenever you enter wilderness areas, there are always some risks. You can protect yourself by being mindful of where you pitch your tent, not sleeping on the ground, keeping food in containers, and being alert for evidence of mice in the area.

- The most common cause of acquisition of the bacterium tularemia is from direct contact with blood or flesh of wild rabbits. Tularemia skin disease in humans is most similar to cat scratch disease, but more severe. Another way to contract tularemia is by inhaling contaminated aerosolized bacteria generated during skinning of animals. Because the tularemia bacterium has high infectivity potential, it can cause a deadly pneumonia. Because it can spread easily through the air, there is concern that it could become an effective bioterrorism agent.

- Another emerging disease of wildlife is chronic wasting disease (CWD), which is a contagious animal neurological disease affecting deer, elk, and moose. It is caused by transmission of prion-associated proteins. These proteins are not even alive, nor do they have nucleic acid building blocks of DNA or RNA. They cause a spongy degeneration of the brain resulting in wasting, abnormal behavior, and death.

- This disease is transmissible among animals through saliva and blood and also from contaminated pastures. There is no treatment. Scientists don't know what happens if you eat a piece of venison that is infected with CWD. If you are a hunter, you can have a local wildlife lab test your deer for CWD. Clinical diagnosis relies on special testing of the brain for prion proteins.

- Another prion-associated disease has caused a degenerative neurological disorder in humans: bovine spongiform encephalopathy. This illness was discovered in England in the mid-1990s, with several dozen citizens dying from eating contaminated beef. Cooking meat does not destroy the prions, nor does it reduce the risk of disease acquisition. In 2014, the risk for transmission of CWD to humans was thought to be low.

Farm Animal Diseases

- We consume many farm animal products, such as pasteurized milk and cheese. The CDC deems drinking raw milk as one of the riskiest behaviors for the acquisition of food-borne illnesses. This is because of the range of germs in raw milk—including *E. coli*, salmonella, shigella, campylobacter, and listeria—that are usually killed by pasteurization.

- Another bacterium, brucella, most commonly affects cattle, pigs, sheep, and goats by causing unintended late-term animal abortions. Sometimes transmitted to humans through milk and cheese from an infected animal, brucellosis causes fever and a body-wide illness that can be life threatening.

- The United States has maintained a federal program for the eradication of brucella from domestic livestock for many years. The United States is very near its goal of being brucellosis-free. Since 2001, for the first time, we reached a point of having no cattle herds quarantined. However, there have been rare cases detected in buffalo herds since then.

- According to the U.S. Dairy Association, cattle and bison in infected geographic areas are recommended for vaccination. The vaccine is a live weakened bacterium. Note that imported milk and cheeses have caused cases of brucellosis in the United States.

- Q fever—named for the original disease with an unknown cause first discovered in Queensland, Australia, in 1935—is a worldwide disease caused by an unusual germ, *Coxiella burnetii*. This is neither a virus nor a bacterium. Cattle, sheep, and goats are the primary reservoirs.

- Organisms are excreted in low numbers in milk, urine, and excrement of infected animals. But the transmission potential of this germ is especially high during animal birthing, when the germ can be aerosolized. Humans get infected by inhaling contaminated barnyard dust. Very few organisms are required to cause infection. Veterinarians, farmers, and slaughterhouse workers are particularly at risk.

- In spite of its deadly potential, most human infection is asymptomatic. When humans do become sick, they usually have pneumonia, but the germ has the potential to spread to all body systems and cause life-threatening infections.

Handling the Human and Animal Transmission of Infectious Diseases

- Since the 1800s, scientists have noted the similarity in disease processes among animals and humans. But human and animal medicines were practiced separately until the late 20th century, until links in the epidemiology and abnormal physiology of diseases were recognized to be common.

- Currently, there is an important collaborative worldwide effort by environmental scientists, human physicians, and veterinarians to prevent, control, and eradicate infectious diseases and to improve the health of all species. It's called the One Health Initiative.

- We are now able to appreciate the potential for repetitive patterns of infections to occur among animals, their environments, and human-animal contacts. This paradigm for global health also recognizes that most new human infectious diseases will emerge from animal reservoirs.

- Deliberate human environmental changes has led to increased contact between people, domestic animals, and wildlife. This can affect the ecological balance of species. In these situations, new habitats for viruses, parasites, and their host vectors can provide opportunities for exchange and transmission of diseases. This has the potential to negatively impact the health of each species.

- We have already witnessed this scenario with malaria, Ebola, and HIV. The One Health Initiative will help provide essential information in anticipating and controlling future infectious disease outbreaks, epidemics, and even the next worldwide pandemic.

Suggested Reading

Quammen, *Spillover*.

Questions to Consider

1. If you have pets, what should you be concerned about in terms of diseases they could spread to you, or diseases from wildlife that could be spread to them?

2. What is so important about rabies that so many people have to get shots for prevention? Are you at risk for rabies in your area?

Tick-Borne Diseases: A Public Health Menace

Lecture 12

Tick-borne diseases have now been deemed a serious public health problem in the United States. The incidence of infection is rising and accounts for tens of thousands of cases each year. Ticks are also expanding their ranges into new areas across the country. Ticks are known to be the vector for at least 14 different illnesses, with a wide range of illness, and new tick-borne illnesses are still being discovered. In this lecture, you will learn about several prevalent tick-borne diseases.

Ticks

- Ticks can sense breath and smells, as well as body heat and vibrations, with a special pair of sensory structures known as palps. These enable ticks to detect an approaching host. Then, they place themselves in a convenient place to hitch a ride when the host comes by.

- Ticks insert a small amount of saliva through the skin that has an anesthetic effect so that you don't even feel the bite. Ticks also have a pair of knifelike structures known as chelicerae that cut open the skin and a barbed structure called a hypostome that they insert through this opening.

- There are many diseases that can be transmitted from tick vectors, and there are several different types of ticks that cause diseases in the United States.

Ehrlichia and Anaplasma

- Ehrlichia and anaplasma have similar tick hosts and similar clinical manifestations, but the geographic domains of these two species are somewhat unique in the United States. Ehrlichia is found most commonly in the central Eastern and central Midwest states, and anaplasma is mostly found in the Northeast and Northern central states.

- Both Ehrlichia and anaplasma, which are neither bacteria nor viruses, are intracellular organisms in white blood cells, with Ehrlichia living in macrophages and anaplasma living in neutrophils. Both cause similar clinical symptoms, including fever, headache, and other flulike symptoms. Neurological symptoms can be more severe and even include confusion, mimicking encephalitis, which is an infection of the brain, or meningitis.

- The lone star tick is the primary vector for Ehrlichia, while anaplasma has both the western black-legged tick and black-legged deer tick. The two diseases were not differentiated from one another until 1990.

- Due to the ever-increasing number of vectors like deer and mice, Ehrlichia and anaplasma incidence is increasing in the United States. In temperate climates, cases occur throughout the year, but cases are more common in northern climates from May through August.

- Both pathogens have cell walls but lack certain common cell membrane components, including several sugars. After inoculation, the germs enter the circulation, where they multiply inside the target white cells. They reprogram the host cell mechanisms, similar to viruses. The germs can occasionally cluster together in white cells in the shape of mulberries, forming microcolonies known as morulae. These structures, although rarely visible, are diagnostic of these infections.

- The diagnosis often relies on clinical judgment, because rapid diagnostic tests are often not available and antibody formation may take weeks. One such rapid test is called polymerase chain reaction technology, which amplifies DNA. However, antibody tests to confirm the diagnosis can be done at serial time points—four weeks later, for example—to look for an increase in the antibody immune response.

- Fortunately, treatment with the antibiotic doxycycline, which affects the ribosomal protein synthesis of these organisms, is effective. Because these organisms lack a cell wall, antibiotics that attack the cell wall, such as penicillins, are not effective. The prognosis worsens if treatment is delayed, and therefore it is important that doxycycline be started immediately if the illness is supported by clinical findings.

Lyme Disease

- Lyme disease is the most common tick-borne infectious disease in the United States. It is caused by a spirochete called *Borrelia burgdorferi* through the bite of a specific species of ticks—black-legged deer ticks.

- The tick has to be attached for more than 24 hours to begin transmitting the spirochete, so it's worth checking yourself each time you are in a wooded area so that you can remove ticks as soon as possible. This can also provide reassurance, because if it has been less than 24 hours from your tick exposure, *Borrelia* transmission is unlikely to occur.

- The acute phase of Lyme illness includes symptoms that usually begin 3 to 14 days after infection and include headache, fatigue, fever, and a telltale bull's-eye rash known as erythema chronicum migrans. This rash is found in nearly 80 percent of Lyme cases and can be at one or more locations on the skin. This rash should not be confused with several centimeters of redness that is often produced around the site of the actual tick bite.

- Up to 20 percent of people with acute illness may develop a focal neurological deficit, especially a Bell's palsy of the face, which fortunately is reversible. Mild forms of meningitis that are not fatal can occur. Much more rarely, an abnormally slow heart rate can lead to dizziness and fainting before being diagnosed.

- Some individuals that have been exposed to *Borrelia* never have any symptoms. Up to five percent of residents of certain Lyme-prevalent states may have true positive blood tests but no recollection of illness. Also, up to five percent of patients may also have a false positive test, due to the nonspecific nature of the IgM immune response mounted to any infection, not specifically Lyme. A second confirmatory blood test, known as a western blot test, is used to confirm the first antibody test as being a true positive result.

- Is it possible for someone who was infected with *Borrelia* to have a negative serological Lyme test? Some people who receive antibiotics early in their illness may not develop antibodies until several weeks later, but they almost uniformly will ultimately have a positive test. This is a common misperception of the general public.

- You also may have heard that there may be deficiencies in the blood antibody tests for Lyme, and a negative test does not exclude having contracted clinical Lyme disease. This can become an issue of contention with individuals who believe that they have ongoing symptoms of Lyme illness but lack any serological evidence of infection.

- The infectious disease community holds relatively firm to the position that only patients with documented positive blood tests for Lyme have the possibility of developing late sequelae, or aftereffects, of Lyme, while other advocate groups disagree with this position. Lyme positive test results usually persist for life, and the magnitude of the test result does not correlate with any later symptoms. This makes Lyme disease more complicated to diagnose if individuals are reinfected.

- There are several oral antibiotic treatments, which commonly include doxycycline and amoxicillin. Patients with certain more-severe neurological or heart forms of the illness may require intravenous treatment. In high-risk Lyme areas of the country, single-dose doxycycline prophylaxis has commonly been implemented for patients with tick bites that have been attached longer than 24 hours, and this preventative measure is as effective as 10 days of medication.

- Left untreated, rare patients can develop late manifestations of Lyme, which are mostly caused by a nonspecific, generalized immune over-response. This may include a debilitating arthritis or, rarely, nerve damage. Because these are immune mediated, chronic long-term oral or intravenous antibiotics are not effective and are not recommended.

- There is a canine vaccine for Lyme disease, but there is no human vaccine. Two pharmaceutical companies developed a human vaccine for Lyme disease that was proven to be 50 to 70 percent effective after two doses. However, over time, the number of vaccinations requested fell from an initial 1.5 million to 10,000, and the vaccines were discontinued due to lack of public interest.

- Also, there were some legal disputes where patients claimed they developed autoimmune symptoms from the vaccine itself. This created a disincentive for pharmaceutical production and development, and production was halted. There are some companies in the process of testing new Lyme vaccines, so perhaps it will come back into favor.

- Once you test positive for Lyme, you will likely always test positive for Lyme. While it is recognized that Lyme disease does not reactivate months or years later, reinfection is possible with a new tick carrying borrelia. These cases may be more difficult to diagnose, especially if there is no erythema chronicum migrans rash.

Rocky Mounted Spotted Fever

- Another tick-borne disease is Rocky Mountain spotted fever (RMSF), which is a rickettsial illness. Its name is a misnomer, because the disease can be found in many areas of the United States and much less often in the Rocky Mountains. American and brown dog ticks, and the Rocky Mountain wood tick, are responsible for this disease.

- Unfortunately, it is the most commonly fatal tick-borne disease in the country. Also, it is not unusual to have family clusters of the disease, because families are outdoors at the same time in areas where the ticks are carrying the germ.

Diagnosing Tick Illnesses

- The classic triad for many tick illnesses includes a tick bite, fever, and a distinctive rash. But from what we now know about ticks, it may be difficult to diagnose tick illnesses because either the person doesn't know that he or she was bitten by a tick, or he or she gets ill five to seven days later and doesn't realize that it was due to a tick, or the symptoms resemble many other illnesses and early blood tests in the first week are usually negative.

- For all tick-borne diseases, a history of a known tick bite occurs less than 50 percent of the time. So, we have to take into account epidemiological clues: Does the patient live in or visit an environment where ticks are prevalent, and/or did he or she perform any high-risk activities, such as walking through tall grass or gardening? If a doctor uses his or her clinical and diagnostic skills correctly and starts doxycycline right away, most patients will get better.

Other Causes of Tick-Borne Illnesses

- Tick-borne illnesses can have other causes. Heartland virus is a newly identified phlebovirus that was first isolated in 2009 from two Missouri farmers hospitalized with fever, low white blood cells, and low platelets. Based on the patients' clinical findings and their reported exposures, their illness was suspected to be transmitted by ticks.

- After this discovery, the CDC worked with local health authorities and learned that heartland virus is found in the lone star tick. The disease is relatively rare, but during 2012 and 2013, six additional confirmed heartland virus disease cases were identified.

- Physicians should consider the diagnosis of heartland virus in patients who develop fever with low white blood cells and platelets without a more likely explanation and who have tested negative for Ehrlichia and anaplasma infection, or who have not responded to doxycycline therapy.

- Southern tick-associated rash illness (STARI) is a tick-borne illness without a known cause yet. It is thought to be transmitted by the lone star tick. Those infected develop a bull's-eye rash similar to Lyme disease, but the illness does not respond to the antibiotics used to treat Lyme. Because we haven't yet identified the cause of STARI, there are no tests and no definitive treatments. Currently, there do not appear to be late aftereffects, such as those that may occur with Lyme.

Preventing Tick-Borne Illnesses

- Preventing tick-borne illnesses can be difficult in certain areas, but you can reduce your risks by adhering to the following steps.
  - Avoid direct contact with wildlife.

  - Use insect repellents in heavily wooded and grassy areas.

  - Wear treated clothing. Several companies now make insect-repelling clothing lines that could be useful for hiking in wooded areas. These are usually treated with permethrin, which

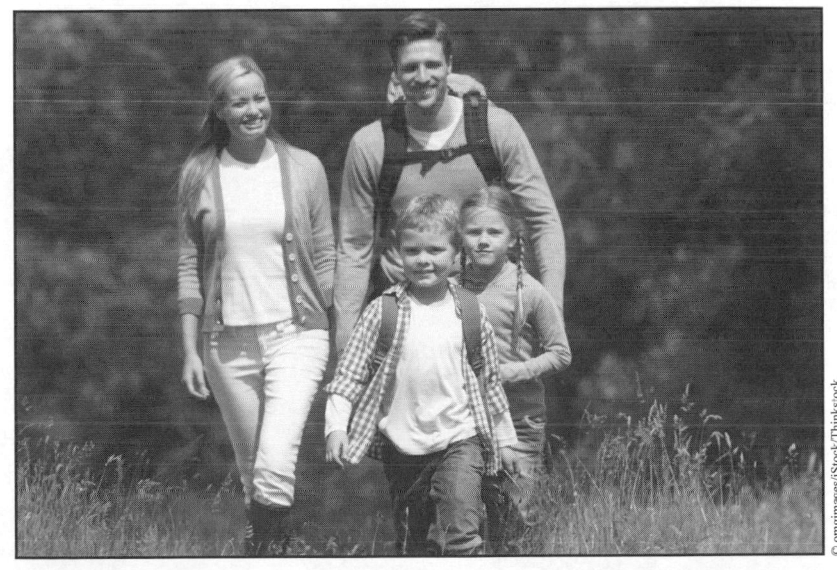

When you are in wooded areas, wear light-colored clothing that covers your body and check for ticks afterward.

has been approved by the Environment Protection Agency for use in clothing.

- Check for ticks after being in areas at risk. If you find one on you that you don't recognize, you can save it in order to identify it through the state health departments.

- Wear light-colored clothing so that you can more easily see ticks.

Suggested Reading

Spreen, *Compendium of Tick-Borne Disease*.

Questions to Consider

1. Why are ticks such a nuisance when it comes to infectious diseases?

2. How can you prevent yourself and family from acquiring tick-borne diseases? Which activities do you do that might put you at risk?

Food-Borne Illness: What's Your Gut Feeling?

Lecture 13

Our guts are a miraculous system of food and nutrient processing, as well as waste disposal, that includes the esophagus, stomach, and duodenum, all the way down through the small and large intestines. When this system is running smoothly, it's like a well-oiled machine; however, when viruses, bacteria, or parasites enter the intestines, it's a whole different story. In this lecture, you will explore gastrointestinal illness, including food-borne illness, travelers' diarrhea, abdominal infection, and a horrible condition called *Clostridium difficile*.

Food-Borne Illness

- Food-borne illness has three major causes: bacteria, preformed bacterial toxins, and viruses. But in 80 percent of cases of food-borne illness, we don't know which of the three is the cause, simply because illness is so common that we can't investigate all of the possibilities. The four most prominent symptoms for gastrointestinal (GI) illness are various combinations of nausea, vomiting, diarrhea, and abdominal pain.

- According to the Centers for Disease Control and Prevention (CDC), 48 million episodes, or 15 percent of all diarrhea in the United States annually, is thought to be due to food-borne disease. This accounts for an estimated 128,000 hospitalizations and 3,000 deaths.

- If you have some combination of the four symptoms, you may have a food-borne illness. All of these symptoms can also be seen in non-food-borne illnesses, including, for example, appendicitis. There are some key questions that will point in the correct diagnostic direction if food-borne illness is suspected, such as the following: What have you eaten in the last 48 hours? How soon after you ate did you feel ill?

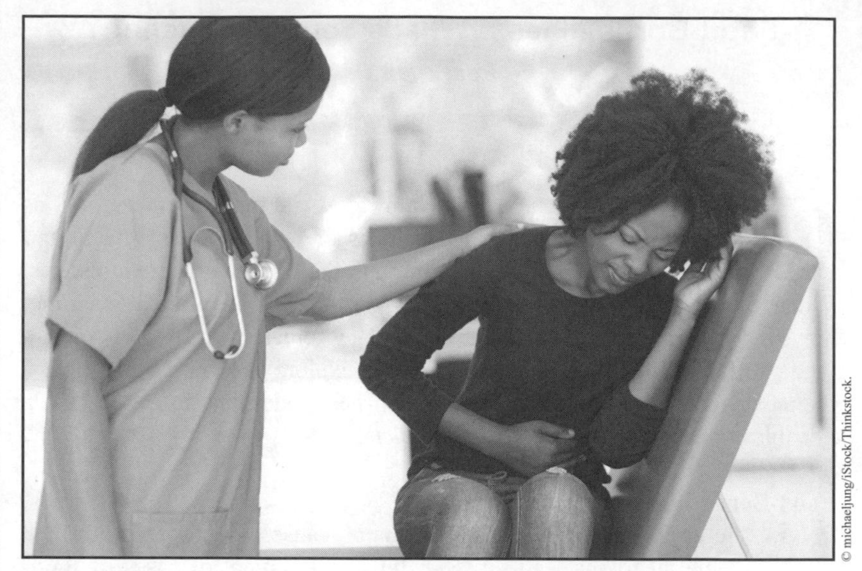

© michaeljung/iStock/Thinkstock.

Gastrointestinal illness occurs when viruses, bacteria, or parasites invade the intestines, resulting in combinations of nausea, vomiting, diarrhea, and abdominal pain.

- If you are sick from something you ate, the general timeline of illness ranges from a few hours to a few days, but epidemiological clues need to be factored into the timeline. When one of the four symptoms presents as the major symptom, it also helps doctors sort out what might be causing the intestinal distress.

Vomiting as the Major Presenting Symptom

- A sudden onset of vomiting and nausea is likely due to the ingestion of a preformed toxin or chemical made by bacteria. Because the toxin is preformed, there is no risk of person-to-person spread. Nausea and vomiting interrupt the normal motility of the GI system. There is a vomiting center, called the area postrema, located in the lower portion of our brain. Input from the GI nervous system from noxious stimuli is transmitted to this brain location. Nausea is likely caused by increased conscious awareness of activity at the vomit center.

- Staphylococcal food poisoning involves the ingestion of a preformed toxin that is not destroyed by heating or rewarming food. No antibiotics are indicated for treatment, and the illness usually resolves within 24 hours.

- Another bacterium, *Bacillus cereus*, also produces a preformed toxin, causing nausea and vomiting. Bacillus is typically found in starchy foods, such as rice. Neither refrigeration nor rewarming affects the toxin.

- With both staphylococcal and bacillus food poisoning, the diagnosis is usually made on clinical grounds—that is, without a lab or blood test—using these criteria: the right opportunity, the right food, the typical illness. Nausea and vomiting are also the predominant symptoms of norovirus infection, which is the most common infectious cause of GI illness in the United States.

Diarrhea as the Major Presenting Symptom

- Diarrhea is defined as an increase in the frequency or volume of bowel movements that are unformed. All diarrhea has one abnormal physiologic event in common: a mishandling of the absorption of water, especially in the colon.

- In addition to norovirus, viral gastroenteritis accounts for another 30 to 40 percent of all infectious diarrhea in the United States. One of the biggest culprits—through the fecal-oral route, or transmission by poor hand-washing and bathroom habits or contaminated water sources—is rotavirus, which is the biggest cause of dehydrating diarrhea necessitating hospitalization in children under age two.

- About three million cases of rotavirus infection occur annually in the United States, mostly from food contamination. The childhood rotavirus vaccine has been shown to be effective in the United States in reducing the burden of this illness by more than 50 percent.

- Worldwide, 800,000 children under five die from diarrhea yearly, which makes diarrhea the second biggest killer of children in the world. For children who become dehydrated, diarrhea could mean the difference between life and death, especially in impoverished areas of the world. The body needs a certain minimum volume of fluid in the arteries and veins to keep the circulatory system pumping and an adequate blood pressure to support the function of major organs, such as the heart, brain, and kidneys.

- Also, diarrhea can cause a major loss of key blood ingredients called electrolytes, especially sodium and potassium. If the sodium and/or potassium levels in the blood becomes too low, muscles do not function well, and there is the potential for abnormal heart rhythms and even sudden death. Rotavirus vaccination in underdeveloped countries is a key goal of the World Health Organization.

Inflammatory Diarrhea as the Major Presenting Symptom

- The presence of white blood cells under the microscope and/or blood in bowel movements defines an inflammatory diarrhea, because the germ is invading the intestinal lining. This shows up in bowel movements as passage of diarrhea with blood or mucus, presence of moderate to severe abdominal pain, and fever.

- There is a wide array of harmful bacteria that cause these symptoms. We are all at risk for invasive food-borne poisoning from the four most common bacteria: salmonella, campylobacter, shigella, and a special type of *E. coli*. Symptoms of all these bacterial diseases may begin as early as 12 hours, but more typically at 48 to 72 hours, after ingesting contaminated food. The bacteria need time to multiply and produce their toxins.

Globalization of the Food Supply

- Where our food is coming from these days is becoming more and more important. Roughly 15 percent of all food consumed in the United States is imported. American consumers want many different kinds of food and expect it to be available year-round. This includes more than 80 percent of seafood and more than 50 percent of fresh produce.

- Foods imported to the United States come from more than 200,000 foreign facilities in more than 200 countries. Many of those foreign food-producing countries may lack food safety standards as strict as those in place in the United States. The rapid globalization of food production increases consumers' vulnerability as well by making any food outbreak harder to trace.

- Traveler's diarrhea is the most common illness in persons traveling from developed to developing regions of the world. About 50 percent of travelers develop diarrhea. Most episodes occur between 4 and 14 days after arrival. Traveler's diarrhea is nearly always benign and self-limited. However, the dehydration that can occur may be severe and pose more of a challenge than the illness itself.

- The reasons are similar to those for rotavirus. The most common germ is yet another species of *E. coli*, known as enterotoxigenic *E. coli*. Travelers should also be aware that food items on aircraft are usually obtained at the city of departure.

- The treatment of traveler's diarrhea includes three different approaches: fluid replacement, meaning that you should keep yourself well hydrated with bottled drinks, especially if you can use rehydration solutions that contain sodium and potassium; antimotility agents, such as Imodium or Pepto-Bismol, which can slow down the volume of fluid loss by acting on the nerve receptors of the intestines; and sometimes antibiotics, if necessary, but not commonly.

- Antibiotics are usually prescribed under the guidance of a travel clinic. They may be warranted for treatment in travelers who develop moderate to severe diarrhea. However, it's important to know that medical help may be needed if you develop a high fever, worsening abdominal pain, and/or bloody diarrhea.

Common Infectious Diseases of the Intestinal Tract

- Common infectious diseases of the intestinal tract include appendicitis, diverticulitis, and *Clostridium difficile*. The appendix is a nonessential organ located in the lower-right quadrant of the abdomen. Blockage, or obstruction of the opening, of the appendix leads to bacteria becoming trapped inside. This leads to inflammation and infection and right-sided lower abdominal pain. Appendicitis in older individuals is usually more serious than the young because 60 to 90 percent are found to be ruptured at the time of surgery.

- What is diverticulitis? In the distal colon, outpouchings known as diverticuli are common. These diverticuli occur in approximately 30 percent of the population over the age of 45 and 60 percent of those over the age of 70. It is estimated that 10 to 20 percent of people with diverticuli will develop an infection when bacteria get trapped, similar to an appendicitis. Ruptures can also occur. Presenting symptoms are similar to those for appendicitis, but on the left side.

- However, unlike appendicitis, diverticulitis can usually be managed conservatively with antibiotics and without surgery. However, if perforation leads to large abscesses, or if the disease recurs frequently, surgery may be necessary. Both of these conditions occur because our own normally good bacteria end up in the wrong place at the wrong time.

- When your gut gets overrun with bad bacteria, you could end up with *Clostridium difficile*, which is an anaerobic, gram-positive, spore-forming, toxin-producing germ. Now listed by the CDC as one of the top emerging infectious disease threats, *Clostridium difficile* can be the cause of antibiotic-associated colitis and can be life threatening.

- Antibiotic use is the most widely recognized and modifiable risk factor for this disease. This is one reason that we don't want to overuse antibiotics unnecessarily. Exposure to health-care environments likely increases the risk of acquiring the germ.

- What happens next to cause disease? Alteration of normal intestinal bacteria due to antibiotic therapy allows this germ to overgrow, with patients having diarrhea of increased intensity and severity. *Clostridium difficile* is capable of elaborating toxins that bind to the surface of intestinal cells. This leads to inflammation, the formation of pus, and watery diarrhea. Outside the colon, it survives as spores, which are resistant to destruction. Once spores are in the colon, they can convert to bacterial forms that produce toxins.

- Dramatic increases, at least a doubling, in the incidence and severity of health-care–associated *Clostridium difficile* infection have occurred since 2000, particularly in patients over the age of 65. Even if the condition is successfully treated with special antibiotics, up to 25 percent of patients may have recurring symptoms weeks later, with 10 percent of these relapsers having another occurrence.

- A new treatment for this condition is known as fecal microbiota transplantation, which takes a healthy person's intestinal microbiota and transplants it into the afflicted patient, with the hope that this will repopulate the intestines with appropriate bacteria to restore a healthy state. In some cases, it has turned around patients with multiple recurrences in a matter of hours, after being extremely ill for weeks. This procedure has approximately a 90 percent success rate.

Suggested Reading

Morris and Morris, *Foodborne Infections and Intoxications*.

Questions to Consider

1. Why are food-borne diseases such a nuisance?

2. What safety measures can you implement to reduce the risk of food-borne disease at home? What if you're going to travel?

Respiratory and Brain Infections

Lecture 14

In this lecture, you will learn about infections of two different organ systems: the respiratory tract and central nervous system. A common thread between these organ systems is their propensity for infectious diseases to become deadly. You will learn how complicated respiratory infections can be and how deadly severe pneumonia and bacterial meningitis can become. In addition, you will learn how to recognize the symptoms of pneumonia and meningitis and when to seek medical attention.

Pneumonia

- Some pneumonias can be contracted by directly breathing in droplets contaminated with aerosolized bacteria. This is one reason that hotels, but especially hospitals, need to pay strict attention to water quality in showers, pools, air-conditioning systems, and hot tubs.

- Legionella bacteria, when aerosolized, can cause pneumonia. The mucous membranes of the throat and respiratory tract are very important in stopping inhaled substances from entering our lungs. However, if you have a chronic lung condition, or if you smoke regularly, these membranes and attached cilia are damaged and can't provide their innate immunity properly. Legionella bacteria can then make their way deeper into the lungs and enter the alveoli, balloon-like structures that help us exchange oxygen. The bacteria continue to multiply in the alveoli, causing pneumonia—an invasion of the alveoli and adjacent lung tissue.

- While failure of the respiratory defenses is common in individuals with the underlying lung disease, you don't need to have abnormal lungs to develop pneumonia. The common physiology of almost all pneumonia is what is known as aspiration from mouth, throat, and teeth bacteria, via gravity, into the lungs. This has nothing to do with inhaling bacteria like legionella.

- Starting innocently in the respiratory tract, the bacteria leads us through twists and turns, ending up in the central nervous system, where it threatens to cause death. Normal bacteria colonize the back of the throat and usually don't cause any mischief.

- One of these is called *Streptococcus pneumonia*, which should not be confused with the Group A streptococcus, which causes sore throats and rheumatic fever. In fact, the most common pneumonia in adults is *Streptococcus pneumonia*. This germ has several means to elude our normal defenses, especially a very thick sugar capsule that makes it difficult for our macrophages to swallow the bacteria. In addition, there are more than 20 different variations on this sugar capsule, and we need specific immunity to each one to protect us from most strains of *Streptococcus pneumonia*.

- If *Streptococcus pneumonia* gets past the upper and lower respiratory defenses, it will cause pneumococcal pneumonia. By that point, the bacteria are fiercely multiplying in the alveolar space. After a certain critical number of bacteria is reached, the person starts to become ill with fever and has increased difficulty breathing and a cough. If the cough is strong enough, it can force out a sputum specimen that can be examined under the microscope to determine the cause of pneumonia.

- It is at this point that the patient will likely seek medical attention. The health-care provider will listen to the patient's lungs and hear abnormal sounds, especially decreased breath sounds in the area of the lung that is filling with white blood cells and other inflammatory cells to fight the pneumococcus. A chest X-ray will show that the normal X-rays that pass through the air in the lung are now blocked by this inflammatory response, and the X-ray will be abnormal with a white zone that defines the pneumonia.

- If medical attention is sought at this point, there is a good probability that the infection can be managed with supportive care and an appropriate antibiotic targeting pneumococcus. Patients can be discharged home with careful medical follow-up with a mortality rate of only 1 percent. Sometimes, depending on the severity of illness, the patient's age, or social factors, hospitalization may be required. The mortality rate for patients hospitalized with community-acquired pneumonia is 12 percent.

- If medical attention is not sought, it is likely that the infection will become more severe and develop into a body-wide, systemic infection. The most common cause of invasive, body-wide infections for people of age 65 and older is invasive pneumococcal disease. This is why it's important to get pneumococcal vaccines if you're 65 or older.

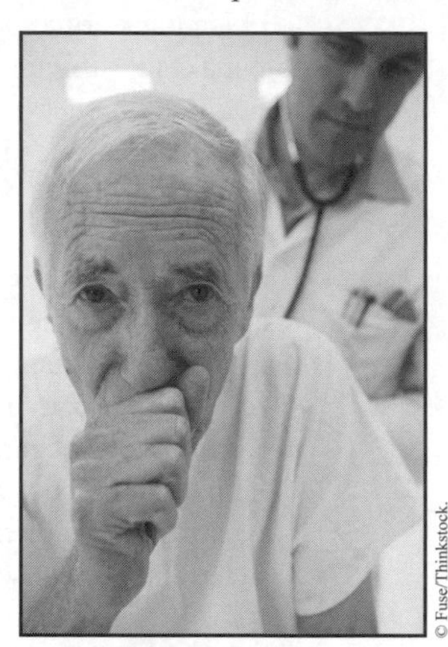

Pneumococcal disease affects the lungs, making it difficult to breathe. Pneumococcal vaccines are especially important for elderly populations.

- The situation can get even worse. As pneumococcus creeps out into the bloodstream, it initiates a more advanced inflammatory process called sepsis, at which point the mortality rate climbs to 40 percent. Additionally, the pneumococcus has a propensity to attack the linings around the brain and spinal cord, causing a condition known as bacterial meningitis, which can lead to impairment in the patient's ability to communicate and, if severe enough, a coma.

- When the infection reaches this dangerous threshold, the patient's life is in jeopardy. The inflammatory response in the lung may be serious enough that the patient may even require the assistance of a breathing machine to provide extra oxygen support to improve the chances of survival. Even though the antibiotics may be working, the inflammatory response in the blood may lead to multiple organ system damage.

- Not all cases of pneumonia, even bacterial pneumococcal pneumonia, end up becoming this serious. There are many other bacterial germs that can cause pneumonia and many other viruses, such as influenza—as well as organisms in between, such as *Mycoplasma pneumonia* or *Chlamydia pneumonia*—that can make us sick.

- There are two vaccinations for *Streptococcus pneumonia* that are available: a conjugate vaccine with 8 to 13 pneumococcal capsule sugar types and another vaccine that is intended to recognize 23 different capsule types of pneumococcus. It is recommended that children receive the conjugate vaccine in the first years of life, and it is recommended that all adults now receive both types of vaccine once after the age of 65. Some individuals with certain chronic medical conditions, especially of the heart or lung, need to receive these vaccinations at least once before the age of 65 as well.

- There are limits to the efficacy of the vaccinations. Not all sugar capsule types are captured with the vaccines, although they are intended to capture about 85 percent of the types causing invasive disease. In addition, your body's individual immune response may result in antibody production for some of the serotypes in the vaccine, but not all of them.

- It is still estimated that the standard 23-valent pneumococcal vaccine leads to a risk reduction of illness of about 50 percent. With the addition of the conjugate vaccine recommendations, the risk of acquiring pneumonia should become even lower.

- You should still seek medical attention for what might be pneumonia and not believe that you are invincible just because you received the vaccination. The same principle holds true for the yearly influenza vaccine.

Meningitis

- Most conditions that cause fever, headache, and a stiff neck—symptoms of meningitis—are not due to a bacterial cause and are usually not life threatening. This medical condition is known as aseptic meningitis. The main cause is usually the result of a viral infection, and while it may not be as severe as bacterial meningitis, it can still make you feel miserable for five to seven days.

- Eighty percent of aseptic meningitis cases are caused by enteroviruses, which cause intestinal symptoms to start but then travel through the bloodstream to the meninges, or membranes that surround the brain and spinal cord, where it can cause meningitis.

- Enteroviruses belong to the family of viruses that includes poliovirus, echovirus, and Coxsackie virus. A similar type of inflammatory response in the meninges is invoked by the immune system for these viruses, although it's typically not as severe.

- Fortunately, our body is usually able to overcome the viral infection without serious consequences. There are no antiviral medications that can be used for most viral meningitis, and vaccination efforts are only beginning for enteroviruses. On very rare occasions, the virus can invade the brain tissue, causing encephalitis, and the illness is more severe with signs of altered consciousness or coma.

- One of the animal, or zoonotic, infections transmitted from robins to mosquitoes to humans, known as West Nile virus, can cause encephalitis. Herpes simplex viruses that usually move forward to cause fever blisters can travel backward toward the spine and cause aseptic meningitis or, uncommonly, encephalitis. Aseptic meningitis can also occur from some of the tick-borne diseases, especially the Lyme spirochete, *Borrelia burgdorferi*. So, if you have a tick bite and you have a severe headache and stiff neck, it is most likely that you have aseptic meningitis.

- It's very important to know the symptoms of infections around the brain and spinal cord so that you can act quickly. The need for medical attention should not be minimized. Although the odds are in your favor that an unusually severe headache is not life threatening, you should not make that determination on your own.

Seek medical attention for a complex of symptoms that combines fever, severe headache, irritation of vision with bright lights, and a stiff neck or back.

Other Upper Respiratory Tract Infections

- There are several sinuses in the front of the face, which also connect with the respiratory passages of the nose and back of the throat. A viral infection causes thickening of respiratory and sinus mucosa, as well as a loss of cilia clearance mechanisms.

- But the illness is usually always viral for the first 10 to 14 days, and the treatment is control of the symptoms and not antibiotics. All too often, at the first sign of a runny nose and congestion leading to pressure over the front of the face, a phone call is placed to primary care providers' offices requesting antibiotics for an infection.

- The official recommendation of the Infectious Disease Society of America and of the American Academy of Otolaryngology is initially not to treat sinus irritation with antibiotics. There are, of course, exceptions that might need antibiotics earlier, including symptoms suggesting early bacterial infections—such as fever more than 101 degrees with severe pain—but these symptoms are not the norm. With all the drug-resistance issues, the less you and your family take antibiotics, the better.

- Bronchitis is another upper respiratory infection. The bronchi are the airway tubes between the mouth and the lower lungs. They can also be affected by infectious organisms in a manner similar to the ears and the sinuses.

- Rhinovirus, or the common cold, is the most common infectious disease condition in the United States. These viruses have a propensity to attack the mucous membranes of the nose, throat, and especially the bronchi.

- It's not unusual to have nasal-congestion symptoms a few days before complaining that you now have a chest cold, manifested by a clear and usually nonproductive cough, which sometimes keeps you awake at night unless you sit in an upright position.

- Bronchitis—except for patients with chronic lung disease, such as emphysema—is exclusively a viral illness and does not require antibiotics.

- Symptomatic care of your cough, likely with decongestants and over-the-counter cough suppressants, is the recommended treatment for bronchitis. It will still be a nuisance and last a week to 10 days, but unless you have symptoms that would suggest you are getting bacterial pneumonia, antibiotics won't help you.

Suggested Reading

Marrie, *Community-Acquired Pneumonia*.

Questions to Consider

1. What does it mean to really have pneumonia, and what kinds of germs cause this condition? What's all the fuss about needing to get a pneumonia vaccine?

2. If you become ill with a fever and a headache, what other symptoms should make you seek medical attention for meningitis, or inflammation of the nervous system? Is all meningitis deadly?

Flesh-Eating Bacteria and Blood Poisoning

Lecture 15

This lecture will continue the examination of infections by organ systems—specifically, infections involving the skin and bloodstream. You will learn how seemingly benign infections in the skin can turn deadly. You will learn about the powerful sepsis syndrome, which is responsible for approximately 10 percent of all the deaths that occur in the United States, as well as approximately 10 percent of all admissions to hospital intensive care units. In addition, you will learn about infections of the lymphatic system, MRSA, and endocarditis.

Skin Bacteria and Infections

- Bacterial infections can wreak havoc with all layers of skin. For example, the top layer of human skin, the epidermis, is covered by millions of bacterial germs, the most common of which is *Staphylococcus epidermidis*. We all have this germ. Unlike its cousin *Staphylococcus aureus*, *Staphylococcus epidermidis* usually lives on the skin without causing disease. But at any moment in time, 30 percent of us also carry *Staphlococcus aureus* on our skin. And at any point in time, about 5 percent of us carry streptococcal germs that could cause skin infections.

- No matter how frequently we shower or bathe, there are always residual bacteria that stick to the top layer of the skin. Cleaning the skin does result in numerical reductions in surface bacteria, but within hours, the bacteria will replicate to reach their normal levels. Each of us has our own natural equilibrium of skin bacteria.

- One example of an infection of the epidermis is called folliculitis, which is an inflammation of follicles, especially hair follicles. Another infection of the epidermis, acne, is a common occurrence. Because the face is a highly vascular area with many pathways to the deeper parts of the brain, resist the temptation to squeeze a pimple on your face.

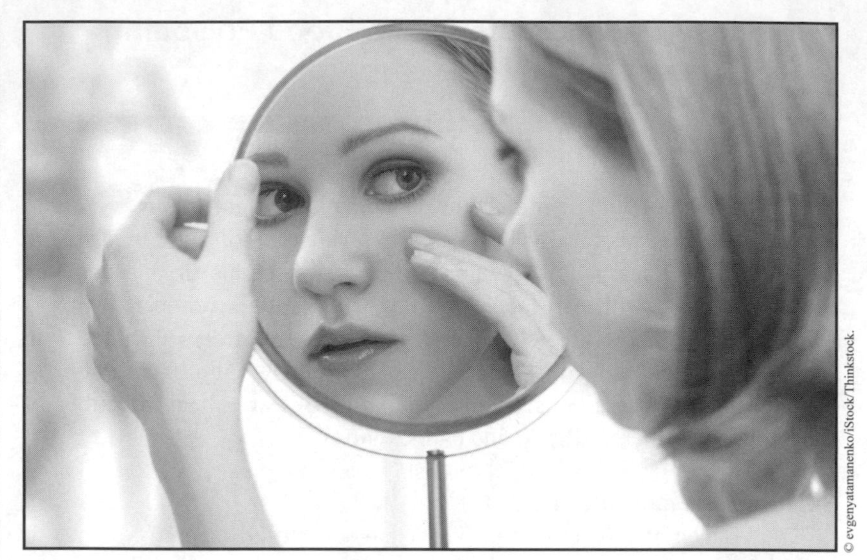

© evgenyatamanenko/iStock/Thinkstock.

Although acne is a common infection of the epidermis, try to resist the urge to squeeze any pimples that might appear on your face.

- Infections that extend slightly deeper into the skin, into the dermis layer, are known as skin abscesses, furuncles, or carbuncles. Typically, these infections begin as folliculitis in the epidermis layer, but the process then extends into the next layer of the skin.

- Most of these infections can be managed with hot compresses, which increase the circulation to the area and enhance the body's normal inflammatory response. If the abscess is large, a minor surgical procedure known as incision and drainage may be required.

- Most skin abscesses also do not require antibiotic therapy. If the diameter of the redness from one side of the abscess to the other is less than five centimeters, then antibiotics are usually not required. A topical antibiotic could be considered.

- For all infections of the skin, it is important to know that bacteria cannot penetrate through intact skin. Hence, there has to be a portal of entry for bacteria to enter the surface or deeper layers of the skin. Often, it may just be a hair follicle or a minor scratch.

- Another skin infection is known as cellulitis. When this occurs, the infection is larger than five centimeters and extends above and below the area that would have been the presumptive portal of entry. It usually is hot, thickened, painful, and very red and can spread to the bloodstream and lymph nodes. *Staphylococcus aureus* and streptococcal germs are the most common culprits in cellulitis. Another example is erysipelas of the face, which is caused by streptococcal germs.

Lymphatics

- Anatomically, within the dermis layer of the skin are also channels of the body that help return extra fluid to the heart. This is known as the lymphatic system. Think of the lymphatic system as a giant spider web over your body that slowly helps move any fluid that is outside of your arteries and veins back to the heart. The fluid is clear and yellow in color and resembles the fluid from the inside of a simple blister.

- Aside from channeling fluid, the lymph system also aids our immune system in transporting necessary components to help fight infection. The lymph system channels into lymph nodes, which is why lymph nodes are enlarged when there is any type of infection. When the lymphatic system is involved with infection—often with an abscess nearby—there is visible red streaking of the skin, known as lymphangitis.

- All cellulitis and lymphangitis will require either oral or intravenous antibiotics, or both, depending on the health-care provider's assessment of the severity of the infection. Puncture wounds of the hands and feet, as well as animal bites, are also forms of cellulitis and lymphangitis. However, under these circumstances, it's the bacteria from the object that causes the puncture, such as bacteria in a dog's or cat's mouth, that are the infection culprits, rather than your own skin bacteria.

- The worst type of skin infection involves all layers of the skin, leading to destruction and essentially death of the skin tissue and muscle. The common term for this is flesh-eating bacteria, but the medical name is necrotizing fasciitis. Although this can be caused by *Staphylococcus aureus* or strep, there are other bacteria that alone, or in combination, that can lead to this condition.

- The management of necrotizing fasciitis is challenging. Virtually all patients have a body-wide sepsis response, which requires control of the infection, antibiotics, and intensive care. Necrotizing fasciitis is considered a medical emergency, and surgery is always required. Multiple surgeries, and even amputation, may be necessary—not only to control the infecting bacteria, but also to remove tissue that is no longer alive.

MRSA

- Methicillin-resistant *Staphylococcus aureus* (MRSA) has been singled out by the Centers for Disease Control and Prevention as one of the most important resistant bacteria of the present day. The original strains of MRSA date back nearly 40 years, to the hospital setting. Staph bacteria acquired a large extra-chromosomal genetic element known as a plasmid, making it resistant to all antibiotics, with the exception of the antibiotic vancomycin.

- The current concerns about MRSA focus on a slightly different variety of MRSA, called community-based MRSA. This organism appeared in the late 1990s and generally has continued to increase in prevalence in the community. It has a smaller resistance plasmid, so there are more antibiotics that can be used for treatment when compared to the hospital strain of MRSA.

- MRSA is present in one percent of the general population but has a prevalence of five percent or more in other special population groups. These groups tend to involve crowded living circumstances, such as inner-city populations or prison inmates, but can also occur as outbreaks among athletic teams. Crowding promotes closer person-to-person skin contact.

- MRSA is not necessarily any stronger or more virulent than regular *Staphylococcus aureus*, but because it is resistant to many common antibiotics, it is more difficult to treat and more likely may require intravenous therapy. Anyone can acquire the germ, because it's spread by skin-to-skin contact or contact with infected surfaces. The most common presentations of community-based MRSA are skin infections, typically carbuncles or boils.

- But simply having the germ on your skin does not automatically mean that you will have problems with infections. An infection may never occur, and the germ may be replaced by normal bacteria of the skin over time. Other people may have a single episode of a skin infection.

Sepsis

- Bacteria in the blood is called bacteremia, or called blood poisoning, and when the bacteria initiate a serious immune inflammatory response, the condition is known as sepsis. When this happens, it can lead to leaky blood vessels and clots. This can impair blood flow and damage the major organ systems to the point where the patient dies.

- Sepsis is a syndrome, not a specific clinical entity, that is part of a broader entity known as systemic inflammatory response syndrome (SIRS). To meet the criteria for SIRS, a patient needs to have the following.
  - Temperature greater than 101 or less than 96 degrees.

  - Heart rate greater than 90 beats per minute.

  - Respiratory rate greater than 20 breaths per minute.

  - White blood cell count greater than 12,000 or less than 4,000, where 10,000 is normal.

- To have sepsis, the cause of the SIRS has to be due to infection. When the systolic, or top, blood pressure number is measured below 90, the condition is further defined as septic shock. In spite of correct antibiotic treatment, death may occur, because infections are complicated by dysfunction of our body organs, including the brain, heart, lungs, and kidneys.

- Invading germs do not cause septic shock by themselves. Infection triggers physiological changes that result in a complex and dynamic interplay of chemical mediators, or cytokines. It is the balance between pro-inflammatory and counter anti-inflammatory events that determines the clinical outcome. In general, pro-inflammatory responses are directed toward eliminating the germs responsible for collateral tissue damage; anti-inflammatory responses attempt to limit tissue injury but may reduce the ability to fight off the germs.

- Both staphylococcal and streptococcal bacteria, or toxin production from either, can initiate sepsis. Specific bacteria may be more likely to cause sepsis than others. For example, *Staphylococcus aureus* in the blood is much more dangerous than *Staphylococcus epidermidis*.

- When gram-positive bacteria are involved, parts of the cell-wall components, such as peptidoglycans, are responsible for inducing a septic response. Gram-negative bacteria have a different cell-wall component, endotoxin, containing lipid A, which triggers this response.

- Paradoxically, antibiotics used for gram-negative bacteria can release more endotoxin as the bacteria are being destroyed. Higher levels of endotoxin are associated with worse patient outcomes. When these microbial triggers are recognized by the immune system, activation of both inflammatory and anti-inflammatory immune mediators, known as cytokines, occurs.

- Two of the first cytokines to be implicated in sepsis were tumor necrosis factor (TNF) and interleukin-1 (IL-1). There are many more. Both are involved in local inflammation, white blood cell recruitment, and the generation of fever. Higher levels of these two circulating cytokines showed a correlation with worse outcomes.

Blocking the effects of IL-1 and TNF in animal models of sepsis led to improved outcomes.

Endocarditis

- A special case of bloodstream infection known as endocarditis is an infection of the inner layer of the heart. The heart normally has four chambers, which are separated from one another by four heart valves that control the flow of blood between the different chambers. When germs invade the blood, they have the ability to latch on to any of the heart valves and start an infection of the heart. Some bacteria are much more adept at this task than others, and *Staphylococcus aureus* is one of those bacteria.

- Once the germs have attached themselves to the heart valves, they start to grow exponentially and, left untreated, may destroy your heart valves and damage heart tissue. Eventually, individuals become ill and seek medical attention, and a diagnosis can be made by culturing the blood for bacteria. It may take four to six weeks before the medical suspicion is high enough to even get blood cultures performed to make a diagnosis.

- You would think that if there is a germ in the blood that you should be very ill, but nature has a number of insidious bacteria that can slowly progress their disease process. Most heart infections are called subacute bacterial endocarditis for this reason.

- If you have a heart valve defect, a dentist may ask you if you have taken your antibiotics before he or she works on your teeth. This is because you can virtually guarantee that the process of teeth cleaning leads to a transient jump of bacteria from the mouth into the bloodstream. This creates a perfect opportunity for these germs to seed an abnormal heart valve and cause endocarditis weeks later. The same logic may apply to people with artificially implanted joints. Taking antibiotics an hour before surgery or dental work will reduce this risk.

Suggested Reading

Hall and Hall, *Skin Infections*.

Vincent, Carlet, and Opal, *The Sepsis Text*.

Questions to Consider

1. How can you get a skin infection or cellulitis? What's all the fuss about methicillin-resistant staphylococcal germs, and what does the term "flesh-eating bacteria" really mean? What will you do to prevent your risk of contracting any of these?

2. What does it mean these days to have blood poisoning, and what is sepsis?

STDs and Other Infections below the Belt

Lecture 16

In this lecture, you will learn about the complex mix of organs involved in sexually transmitted diseases and other infections, which involve the urinary tract system, prostate gland, and reproductive organs. You will learn about the many nuances of urinary tract infections and the sometimes complex and controversial topic of sexually transmitted diseases, including chlamydia, genital herpes, and HPV. Even if you are a monogamous adult who has been married for years, sexually transmitted diseases could affect you in several ways, besides the obvious public health impact and associated health-care costs.

Urological Infections

- Nearly every woman has had a bladder infection, otherwise known as cystitis, sometime in her life. The bacteria found near the female urethra are similar to those near the rectal area, which has a supply of germs ready to cause an infection. Because the female urethra is short relative to males, it's easier for bacteria to gain access into the female urethra.

- *E. coli* is notorious for being the cause of bladder infections. It has a structure known as pili that are adapted to holding onto any skin cells that have minor disruptions to their surfaces. This is particularly common in the vaginal area of estrogen-deficient older women.

- Once bacteria attach to the urethral area, they can advance into the bladder—the precursor to an infection known as bacterial cystitis. In order to cause a true infection, the bacteria must invade the inner surface of the bladder wall, and the body's immune response will be triggered to attract white blood cells.

- The presence of bacteria in the urine, however, does not necessarily mean that there is a urinary tract infection. Sometimes bacteria can learn to exist harmoniously in the bladder, without actually causing an infection, a condition known as asymptomatic bacteriuria.

- If you are seeing your health-care provider with no symptoms of a bladder infection, but a collected urine sample shows bacteria on a urinalysis—or, even worse, the provider cultures the urine just to see if there are bacteria present—then you don't need antibiotics. Asymptomatic bacteriuria also exists in older men, but the prevalence of bacteriuria is lower.

- Why should you potentially refuse antibiotics? There have been multiple long-term studies showing that there is no decrease in kidney function or increase in mortality associated with bacteriuria, even if you have diabetes. When there is a real bladder infection, more than 90 percent of cases of cystitis will have symptoms that are all too familiar to women: urinary frequency, urgency, burning or pain with urination, discomfort over the bladder, and often blood in the urine. For bladder infections, your body temperature may be elevated, but fever is rarely greater than 100.5 degrees, a borderline fever.

- A more complicated situation exists in assisted-living facilities and nursing homes. The medical personnel are almost uniformly taught that any change in an individual's cognitive status is automatically due to a urinary tract infection. It's true that any infection in the elderly can cause a change in cognition as a manifestation of infection, but this change is nonspecific and should be persistent or worsening before blaming a urinary tract infection, especially without bladder symptoms.

- In a report in the spring of 2014 by the Centers for Disease Control and Prevention on excess use of antibiotics in health-care settings, unnecessary use of antibiotics for presumptive urine infections was the number one cause of overuse—and, therefore, increased the likelihood of antibiotic resistance. They estimated that if prescribed judiciously, there could be a 37 percent reduction in overall antibiotic use.

- Usually, bladder infections in women are uncomplicated and can be treated for three to seven days. Some women may suffer from recurrent symptomatic bladder infections. Although cranberry juice or cranberry pills are safe and have no serious side effects, the evidence from studies is not overwhelmingly positive.

- On some occasions, the bacteria causing a bladder infection can ascend the urinary tract and lead to a kidney infection, a condition known as pyelonephritis. This is usually a more serious medical condition and prompts the need for stronger antibiotics for a longer duration of time, up to two weeks. This condition sometimes might require intravenous antibiotics or even hospitalization. On rare occasions, the bacteria may actually jump into the bloodstream, causing bacteremia and sepsis.

- Usually, kidney infections are accompanied by higher fevers of 101 degrees or greater and associated pain in the back or flank underneath the rib cage. Some elderly individuals may have neither fever nor back pain and still have a kidney infection.

- Men have their own unique infection of the prostate gland, called prostatitis. If bacteria enter the male bladder, they don't have to travel very far to invade the prostate gland. When this occurs rapidly, leading to sudden difficulties in urination and associated pelvic pain, the condition is known as acute prostatitis. An extended course of antibiotics specifically targeted at the unusual acidic environment of the prostate is needed for cure.

- Some men are plagued by relapses of this condition, because not all of the germs may be completely eradicated from the prostate. Some can remain dormant for months or even years before causing recurrent symptoms, leading to a condition known as chronic recurrent prostatitis.

Chlamydia

- The prevalence of the spectrum of sexually transmitted diseases (STDs) in the United States can be viewed as a pyramid, with

HIV infection at the top and genital herpes, the most prevalent, at the bottom. The three most prevalent diseases at the bottom of the pyramid are chlamydia, genital herpes virus, and human papillomavirus.

- Although each has its own unique characteristics, the main symptoms of STDs are similar to bladder or prostate infections: burning on urination due to an infection of the urethra and/or a vaginal, cervical, or urethral discharge. It is highly unlikely that you could get an STD from a public restroom toilet seat, but you can contract STDs through intercourse, oral sex, and skin-to-skin contact with infected sores.

- *Chlamydia trachomitis* is not truly a bacterium or a virus but is instead an in-between germ. Although not the most prevalent, it has the highest yearly incidence of new cases among STDs, with more than one million cases diagnosed in the United States every year. It most commonly affects younger adults who are sexually active but does not show any bias for a specific age.

- Cervical infections in females are often asymptomatic. The worst part about this infection is that it can ascend into the female reproductive system and is the number one cause of female infertility in the United States. This has become so problematic that the U.S. Preventive Health Task Force recommends screening of all adolescents during every routine health-care visit. Fortunately, the testing has become more sophisticated, and a urine sample tested by molecular diagnostic tests is reliable for establishing a diagnosis, rather than invasive pelvic examinations or male urethral swabs.

- Our knowledge of emerging infectious disease issues continues to evolve over time, and new microbes are being discovered at every turn. Fortunately, at this time, chlamydia and the other in-between germs are treatable with antibiotics, including tetracyclines and erythromycin derivatives that target cellular protein synthesis.

Genital Herpes

- Moving next to the bottom of the STD pyramid, herpes simplex virus (HSV) is the most prevalent STD in the United States, affecting 22 percent of the population. This equates to between 45 million and 60 million Americans with genital HSV infections.

- Genital HSV, similar to herpes labialis, is not cleared and remains latent in the pelvic nerves, so it has the highest prevalence—basically, you have it for life. The main worry with this organism is that only 10 percent of individuals actually know that they have acquired the virus.

- If herpes always presented in a typical fashion with multiple, painful genital ulcers, then everybody would recognize it, but because most HSV infections are subtler, most people are unaware that they have been infected. This creates a major problem, because the virus can be highly contagious.

- If the initial genital herpes infection is recognized, then there are painful vesicles, similar to fever blisters or cold sores. The primary episode tends to be the most severe, because the immune system is unprepared for the first event.

- Infected individuals do develop some degree of long-term immune recognition. However, the immune system is imperfect, and recurrences are common. Recurrences are most common within the first year and present as a painful crop of blisters, but fever is uncommon.

- Illness, even with antiviral medication, typically lasts five to seven days. Recurrences can continue to occur throughout an individual's lifetime but are much more common in the first five years after acquisition of the virus. There fortunately are several antivirus medications for herpes that can be used to ameliorate the course of primary disease, treat recurrences, and sometimes even prevent recurrences.

- There are times when herpes virus is actively shed in vaginal or seminal secretions, without the development of visible vesicles on the skin. This accounts for some of the "silent" HSV transmissions.

HPV

- The last STD in the pyramid is human papillomavirus (HPV), which is a ubiquitous virus with an estimated 20 million individuals in the United States currently infected and 6 million newly infected annually. The HPV prevalence among girls and women is 27 percent overall but has its highest prevalence of 45 percent from ages 14 to 26. The prevalence gradually declines with increasing age, because 90 percent of new HPV infections regress over 6 to 18 months.

- Most HPV infections are not only asymptomatic but also are too small to be clinically noticeable. Externally, however, infections can be visible as warts. The most important concern about HPV, however, is that it is implicated in more than 99 percent of cervical cancers. Persistent infection is a prerequisite for progression to cervical cancer.

- There are a large variety of subtypes of HPV, but only a limited number of them are associated with cancer. These are the types targeted in vaccination. Cervical cancer is one of the top 10 causes of female cancer mortality. The HPV DNA can insert itself into the DNA of the host cell. HPV has the potential to cause oncogenes, which lead the host cell to develop malignant characteristics. HPV is responsible for five percent of all cancers in the world, not just cervical cancer, including throat and anal cancer, in both men and women.

- The main reason for women to have a Pap smear of the cervix performed approximately every three years is to screen for cervical cancer. There are now more sophisticated molecular diagnostic tests to look for the higher-risk variants of HPV that are associated with cancerous transformation. These may eventually replace Pap smears.

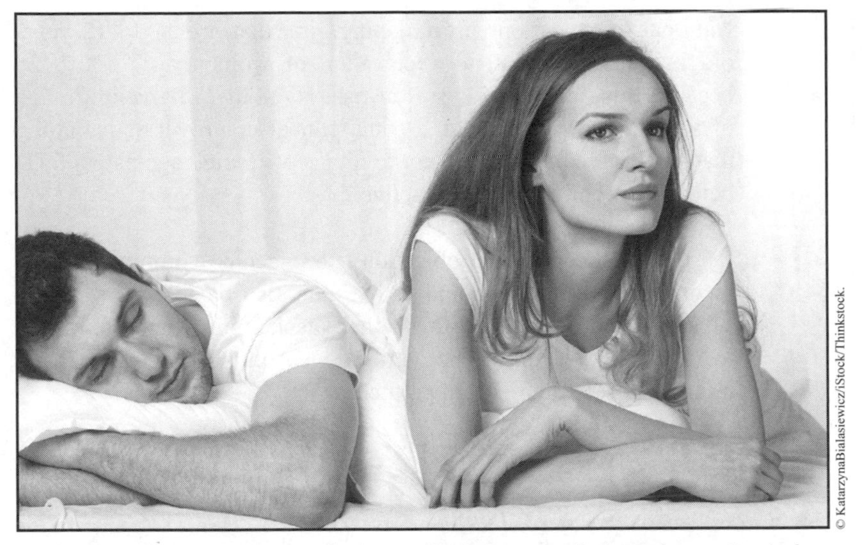

There is a wide range of sexually transmitted diseases that can be contracted through intercourse, oral sex, and skin-to-skin contact with infected sores.

- There are more than 100 types of HPV and 13 types that can cause cervical cancer. About 70 percent of the cervical cancer cases are caused by genotypes 16 and 18, while 90 percent of genital warts are caused by genotypes 6 and 11.

- In 2006, the FDA approved an HPV vaccine for use in females 9 to 26 years of age. This vaccine offers protection from infection for HPV genotypes 6, 11, 16, and 18, which cause the most incidences of cervical cancer and genital warts. A second HPV vaccine was approved in 2009 and contains only genotypes 16 and 18.

- No matter which vaccine is chosen, the vaccines are immunogenic for the creation of antibodies to protect against chronic HPV infection. Immunity is thought to last for at least 10 years, and at the present time, no booster is recommended. The vaccine needs to be administered before exposure to HPV infections, because there is no protection from HPV disease for infections acquired before vaccination.

- National organizations are targeting girls that are 11 to 12 years old but also recommend vaccination of women ages 13 to 26 because this age group is still at risk. Naturally, this youthful age of vaccination has generated some ethical controversy, including that some parents likely object to giving a vaccine against an STD before their child is sexually active.

- In spite of the potential objections, the vaccine committees have recommended that boys and young men also receive the vaccine. This is based on the hypothesis that vaccination would contribute to reduced HPV prevalence among men and, therefore, reduced transmission to their sexual partners.

Suggested Reading

Skloot, *The Immortal Life of Henrietta Lacks*.

Questions to Consider

1. If your doctor tells you that you have a urinary tract infection, but you have no symptoms of irritation, do you really need to take an antibiotic?

2. Are there any long-term consequences of acquiring a sexually transmitted disease in one's youth?

Stay Out of the Hospital!

Lecture 17

This lecture will take you behind the scenes at the hospital, which is perceived as a pristine and sterile environment but is really bustling with all kinds of germs that have the potential to make you and your loved ones sick. You will learn how patients can acquire hospital-based infections, what is being done by the health-care system to prevent them, and what you can do to protect yourself if you are unlucky enough to require hospitalization.

Hospitals

- Hospitals have the advantage of offering specialized care, as well as specialized technologies. If you are ill and need hospitalization, it's great to have a coordinated team of physicians, nurses, and other health-care providers with experience in treating hospitalized patients. Having an experienced trauma team can certainly make the difference between life and death.

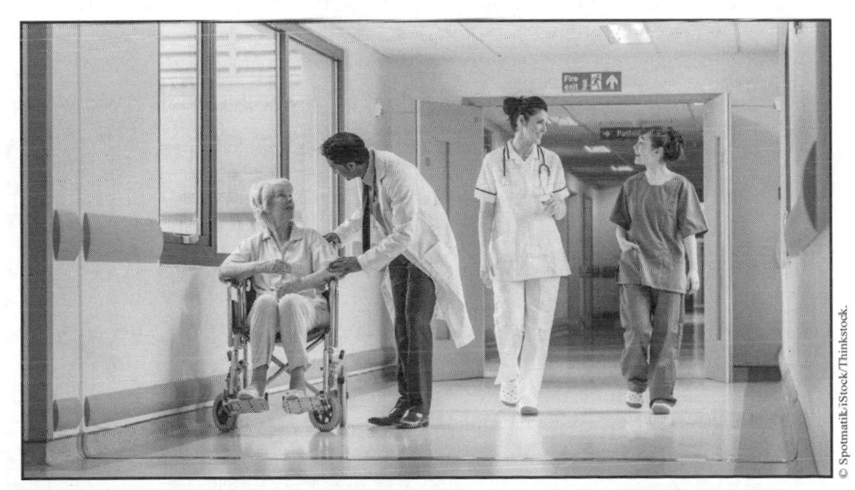

Hospitals are not as sterile as you might think they are; avoid going to the hospital unless you really need to.

- With all these great modern medical resources at our disposal, why is it good advice to avoid being in the hospital unless it is absolutely necessary? There lurks a dark side of the hospital—one in which a patient could actually contract an infectious disease he or she didn't have at the time he or she was admitted. From 2014 national statistics, we know that four percent of patients will acquire an infection after arriving in the hospital.

- Infections acquired in the hospital are known as nosocomial infections. Most nosocomial infections are bacterial, but some can be viral. The major causes are pneumonia, surgical wound infections, and gastrointestinal (GI) infections—each at about 20 percent of the total. Of the pneumonia cases, nearly half are associated with being in intensive care and connected to a breathing machine known as a ventilator.

- Because patients often have catheters placed in their bladders to monitor urine output, or catheters in their arms for intravenous fluids and medications, these anatomical sites are also prone to infection. Each accounts for an additional 10 percent of cases. Pneumonia and bloodstream nosocomial infections have the greatest potential for severe consequences—even death.

- An increasingly important cause of nosocomial GI infection is the bacterial disease known as *Clostridium difficile*. This is the single most common intestinal pathogen, causing 12 percent of all nosocomial infections. *Clostridium difficile* can be transmitted through the fecal-oral route with poorly sanitized hands.

- Resistant bacteria play a more prominent role in nosocomial infections, because the germs have been hanging out in the hospital environment, such as on bedrails, in sinks, and in bathrooms. Some examples include multidrug-resistant gram-negative bacilli and methicillin-resistant *Staphylococcus aureus*.

- The importance of nosocomial infections has always been known to physicians, but the general public was first introduced to these concerns with a report from the Institute of Medicine in 1999. The report concluded that from 44,000 to 98,000 deaths per year in the United States were due to preventable medical errors in hospitals, and a sizable proportion of these were deaths from nosocomial infections.

- By August of 2007, the U.S. government's Medicare, a central health-care agency, said that it would no longer pay for the added cost of certain nosocomial infections, which included catheter-associated urinary tract infections and bloodstream-catheter associated infections. The hospital would have to take medical, legal, and financial responsibility for such infections.

- Hospitals are also now required to report the incidence of catheter-associated urinary tract infections, catheter-associated bloodstream infections, ventilator-associated respiratory events, and surgical wound infection rates to the central health-care agencies and be benchmarked against their peers.

- Teams have been at work at hospitals over the past two decades to reduce the incidence of nosocomial infections. The vast majority of nosocomial infections are device or procedure related. Hospitals have a good grasp of how these infections happen and are actively seeking ways to prevent them, and they are making progress with device-associated infection rates, which have decreased by about 50 percent over the past decade.

- For urinary devices, efforts are focusing on not even placing catheters in the first place — or, if needed, removing them as soon as possible, because the risk of infection is proportional to the number of days the catheter is in place. For pneumonia, there is a bundle of interventions, such as keeping the head of the bed elevated and using special disinfectant mouthwashes to reduce infection risk.

- There are approximately 200 million intravenous catheter devices in use per year in United States and approximately 500,000 device-related bloodstream infections in United States each year, with approximately 25,000 deaths.

- Having a catheter in a vein provides a direct entry route for bacteria to enter the blood. These bacteria can crawl down the side of the catheter into the vein. Alternatively, bacteria can crawl down the inside tunnel of the catheters into the bloodstream. When a vascular catheter is inserted directly into a large blood vessel, the risk of infection is higher than those in the arms.

Preventing Nosocomial Infections

- On a broader scope, in order to prevent all types of nosocomial infections, the Centers for Disease Control and Prevention (CDC) has developed a 12-step plan for preventing infections. The 12 steps are centered on four major principles: preventing transmission, reducing the risk of infection, using antibiotics wisely, and effectively diagnosing and treating infections if they occur.

- First, each hospital, no matter how big or small, has an infection control department. This means that there is an entire health-care team that is looking out for your health in the hospital behind the scenes, in addition to your primary physician. The team includes at least one epidemiologist and one or more nurses to coordinate efforts to reduce infections.

- There are basic infection control principles that health-care providers must follow to protect both you as a patient and themselves from transmittable pathogens. These are known as standard or universal precautions and can be used both to protect health-care providers and for preventing transmission to patients. These measures include hand washing, implementing isolation restrictions, and protecting against blood-borne pathogens with personal protective equipment such as gloves, gowns, and face shields.

- In terms of hand washing, you would think that all physicians and other medical personnel would automatically wash their hands between contact with hospitalized patients, but that's not the reality. Hand hygiene compliance is at best around 90 percent, but more typically in the 70th percentile. Also, nurses, perhaps not unexpectedly, are more judicious about hand washing than physicians, because they are more directly involved with day-to-day patient care.

- There are additional special forms of isolation, including the following.
  - Contact precautions, where providers need to wear gowns and gloves to protect themselves from acquiring germs on their hands or clothes.

  - Droplet isolation, when providers wear a mask. This is used for patients with suspected viral respiratory illnesses, such as influenza.

  - Airborne isolation, where special masks are worn and hospital rooms with special airflow control are needed for diseases such as chicken pox or tuberculosis that can spread beyond six feet.

- The infection control department is responsible for ensuring that the appropriate level of isolation is instituted. For example, a suspected Middle East respiratory syndrome (MERS) case would require airborne and contact isolation from the first suspicion of the disease.

- A special type of isolation is necessary for patients known to be positive for *Clostridium difficile*: enhanced contact precautions. This includes gowns and gloves but also special mandatory soap and water hand washing to remove spores from health-care providers' hands.

- *Clostridium difficile* produces spores that contaminate the hospital environment, such as beds, guardrails, and intravenous pumps. Spores are not only highly contagious but also cannot be killed with alcohol alone—hence the need for soap and water hand washing.

- This introduces yet another dimension of infection control: sterilization and disinfection. When surgery is performed, it is not unusual to enter sterile body spaces, such as the inside of the abdomen. Physicians in the operating room have sterile gloves, a sterile gown, and a mask to prevent them from coughing or sneezing into the wound.

- In terms of instruments in the operating room, there are three types of sterilization that kill both bacteria and spores. Instruments undergo either high-temperature steam sterilization in an autoclave, gas sterilization with low-temperature ethylene oxide gas, or hydrogen peroxide gas plasma.

- Disinfection is one step short of sterilization, and the cleaners used are one of the elements that give hospitals that unique smell: Common bleach, when diluted 1:10 with water and not used directly on the skin, is an excellent disinfectant.

- Another principle of infection prevention is antibiotic prophylaxis in surgery. In nearly all surgery, there is some minor contamination of the wound, no matter how well the surgical site is scrubbed with antimicrobial soap and no matter how careful the surgeons are in operating. So, having antibiotics in the tissues of the surgical wound when that minor contamination might occur has been shown to greatly reduce the risk for most surgical procedures.

- In addition to preventing transmission, another one of the major steps in the CDC program to reduce hospital infections is to diagnose and treat infections effectively. This becomes particularly challenging when we are dealing with diseases that are not mainstream, such as the newly emerging diseases of MERS, SARS, bird flu, etc.

- One of the problems we had when Ebola first entered the United States is that it was not diagnosed correctly right away. Without the correct diagnosis and treatment, many others became exposed, including health workers.

- Also, one of the most difficult decision-making processes for physicians caring for patients with suspected infections is to decide which germs are really causing an infection—versus those just inhabiting their normal environment. Treating bacterial colonization, not infection, is responsible for a large amount of antimicrobial overuse.

- Another CDC initiative is to use antimicrobial agents wisely. Stopping antibiotics when infection is unlikely or cured is essential. Similar to the infection control department, there is a relatively new program for hospitals that has been effective for the past decade known as antimicrobial stewardship, which is responsible for monitoring antibiotic usage.

- The two main goals of antimicrobial stewardship are to eliminate unnecessary antibiotic use and improve the quality of use through constructing hospital guidelines for antibiotic use, restricting last-resort antibiotics to cases that absolutely need them, and educating physicians and other staff about why this is necessary.

- The fourth major component of the CDC program is preventing infection. This requires all medical personnel to proactively anticipate when an infection might occur and reduce its risk—for example, leaving a urinary catheter in place only for short periods at a time.

- The CDC's most recently published Guidelines for Hand Hygiene had two major new recommendations: The first involves using hand sanitizers for routine hand disinfection and only washing with soap and water when hands are visibly dirty, and the second involves establishing monitoring programs for hand hygiene compliance. Using alcohol-based hand sanitizers has enabled hygiene to become more convenient and less time consuming.

- The Joint Hospital Commission, another health-care governing agency, made hand-washing compliance a national patient-safety goal. It requires hospitals that are seeking accreditation to develop both compliance monitoring and improvement programs.

Protecting Yourself in the Hospital

- If you are in the hospital, discourage visits from people who are ill. You can also ask visitors to sanitize their hands and follow hospital isolation precautions when they come into your room. In some instances, they will be asked to wear a gown and gloves. These are simple but effective ways to help control disease spread.

- Everyone who provides care for you should clean their hands. If you do not see your caregivers clean their hands when entering your room, please ask them to do so. We all have a role to play in people staying as healthy as possible when they're in the hospital or even in a medical clinic.

- If you are coming to a medical clinic visit with a cough, asking for and wearing a mask when you are ill and will be in contact with others would be useful. By working together, patients, visitors, and health-care workers can lower the hospital-acquired infection rates. But for now, stay out of the hospital if you can.

Suggested Reading

Nuland, *The Doctors' Plague*.

Weston, *Fundamentals of Infection Prevention and Control*.

Questions to Consider

1. What kinds of infections are lurking in the hospital that you might acquire if you needed to be hospitalized?

2. What do a hospital and medical staff do to try to prevent hospital infections, and how can you help keep yourself safe in the hospital?

The Nemesis of Mankind: HIV and AIDS

Lecture 18

The subject of this lecture is human immunodeficiency virus (HIV), along with the syndrome it causes: acquired immunodeficiency syndrome (AIDS). In this lecture, you will learn how HIV affects the body, why HIV continues to be a worldwide problem, how we are trying to reduce the spread of HIV, and what treatments and vaccines are becoming available. HIV and AIDS will continue to be an elephant on the back of the world as we struggle to control it, but new developments in vaccine development and genetic engineering offer hope.

HIV and AIDS

- More than three decades after the first cases of AIDS were reported, we are still dealing with a pandemic of 33 million people currently with the virus, of which around 3 million are children. There still is no cure, and we have lost nearly 25 million people to the disease. HIV is the number one cause of death in Africa and the leading cause of death from a single infectious disease all over the world.

- Even though the numbers of deaths have declined—partly due to new treatments and prevention—there are more than 6,000 new infections daily worldwide. Even in the United States, there are over a million people living with HIV. These are just the reported cases. Of those in the United States who are infected, around 16 percent don't know they have HIV.

- The incidence of HIV infection in the United States over the past decade has decreased by 33 percent, but one-fourth of new cases of HIV in the United States are of people 13 to 24 years old, and the majority are unaware that they are infected. This has major implications for the country's youth. Unfortunately, only 22 percent of high school students who are sexually active have ever been tested for HIV.

- People are infected by the HIV virus by sharing body fluids, including blood, seminal and vaginal fluids, and even breast milk. If the fluids containing HIV virus come into contact with a damaged mucous membrane or the skin, the virus can enter into the surface cells, and then, over the course of several days, make their way into the bloodstream and spread. HIV can be transmitted by needles—by intravenous drug use, for example.

- HIV is not spread by hugging, shaking hands, sharing dishes or glasses, or using toilet seats. Although it seems logical that HIV could be spread through saliva, the saliva of infected individuals contains only noninfectious components of HIV; saliva also has immune defense properties that disrupt cells that are the actual carriers of the virus. HIV cannot be transmitted through the air, and it does not survive long outside the body.

- The only mandatory testing currently in place is for blood and organ donors, military personnel, some inmates, and newborns in some states. The Centers for Disease Control and Prevention (CDC) does recommend routine HIV screening in primary-care settings for all

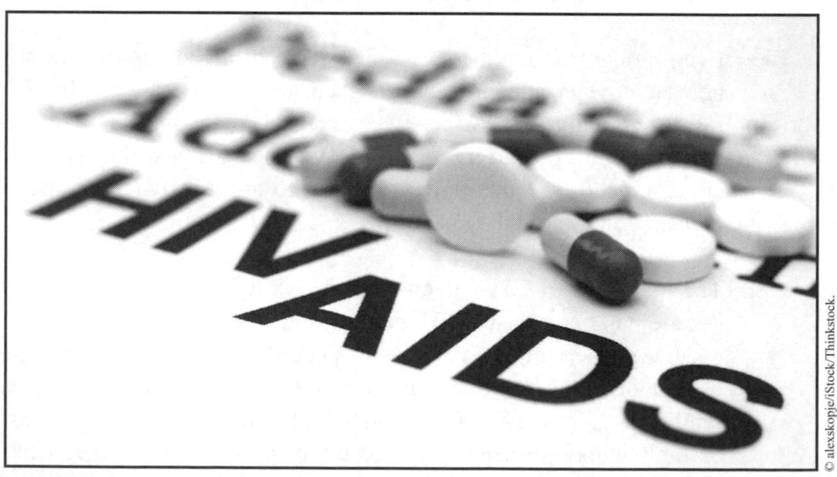

Over the past few decades, there have been pharmaceutical breakthroughs for HIV/AIDS that have resulted in increased quality and length of life for some patients.

adults, ages 13 to 64, once in a lifetime, and repeat screening at least annually for those at high risk. HIV can be transmitted from mother to child during pregnancy, birth, or breastfeeding. Accordingly, the CDC recommends routine testing as part of prenatal care.

The HIV Virus

- Once individuals are infected with the HIV virus, similar to herpes viruses, they are infected for life. The human immune system can't seem to make the virus disappear, because the virus is actually attacking the portion of the immune system that is normally responsible for immune clearance. HIV can hibernate for extended periods of time in the body, but especially in the lymph nodes, bone marrow, and spleen—areas of importance to our immune system.

- The main cells that HIV attacks are the T-helper cells of the immune system, also known as CD4 cells. T-helper cells assist with a larger number of important immune responses of the body. With reduced T-helper CD4 cells, the immune system is handicapped and eventually may be crippled. The HIV virus has the ability to destroy more than a billion CD4 cells daily.

- HIV replication occurs directly in these cells. After the initial infection, the body's production of CD4 cells can compensate for the losses. But, over time, as the HIV destruction process continues, the immune system gradually declines with reduced numbers of CD4 cells.

- HIV is the virus that causes AIDS. But AIDS isn't really a disease; it's a complicated syndrome with many symptoms. AIDS is the last stage of an HIV infection. The immune system is so damaged that people begin to get opportunistic infections, meaning that they normally would not occur with healthy immune systems. Examples of such infections include pneumocystis pneumonia and cryptococcal fungal meningitis.

- Cancers are also much more common with AIDS, including lymphomas and a particularly virulent skin cancer known as

Kaposi's sarcoma. Fortunately, in developed countries with antiretroviral drugs, most patients no longer get to this stage of their illness. With proper treatment, called antiretroviral therapy (ART), patients can usually keep the level of HIV virus low.

- ART is the use of HIV medicines to fight HIV infection. It involves taking a combination of HIV medicines every day. These medications can control the virus so that patients can live a longer, healthier life. ART also reduces the risk of transmitting HIV to others.

- Today, people in developed countries who are treated before the disease becomes advanced can have a nearly normal life expectancy. For example, "Magic" Johnson, former star basketball player, was still healthy more than 20 years after his HIV diagnosis. Deaths from other diseases have surpassed deaths from opportunistic infections in the current ART therapy era.

- No safe and effective cure for HIV currently exists, but scientists are working hard to find one and remain hopeful. Consequently, HIV prevention is paramount.

Pharmaceutical Breakthroughs

- The first drug breakthrough toward managing this terrible disease came when Jerome Horwitz, a scientist studying cancer, developed zidovudine, also known as AZT. In 1964, it was originally designed to be used as a cancer drug, but it was a failure; 25 years later, it was surprisingly found by other scientists to have antiretroviral activity, and it became the first ART medication. This was the first treatment to give hope to HIV patients.

- While AZT was found to be effective, it only made a small dent in a patient's viral burden in the blood. This reduced the viral load by one logarithm—for example, from 1 million down to 100,000 virus particles. Also, when used alone, resistance rapidly developed. In addition, AZT was not without several significant side effects, especially nausea. However, due to the crisis state of the HIV/AIDS pandemic, and for humanitarian reasons, this drug was approved within 20 months, rather than taking the usual 8 to 10 years.

- Because there are between 1 and 10 billion HIV viruses replicating daily, there is a large and rapid turnover of genetic material and, hence, a high probability for the potential of drug-resistant mutant viruses to emerge. HIV reverse transcriptase also has a high error rate in reading its genetic code, so this enhances the potential for mutations and for drug resistance.

- If patients are not adherent to taking all the doses of their medications, this can result in subtherapeutic viral drug levels, which greatly increases the risk of drug mutations. In fact, the odds of being infected with an HIV virus without mutations that encode for drug resistance is becoming increasingly rare.

- Sometimes, mutant HIV virus is not necessarily more virulent. In fact, the mutant virus can be weak enough that it will not have a long-term survival advantage and, hence, becomes clinically insignificant. The capacity for rapid mutations reinforces the need for continued aggressive pharmaceutical development in the field.

- Since AZT, there are now more than 20 ART choices, with several in development and others entering into clinical trials. The estimated treatment cost for a patient infected with HIV is 400,000 dollars or more over a lifetime.

Prevention: U.S. and Global Health Policy

- Because HIV is so difficult to treat once the virus is acquired, and because management requires lifelong attention, the ideal means to manage HIV is through prevention. Because HIV may be transmitted by blood contamination, avoiding blood splatter is common sense. Realistically, HIV acquisition would require an open break in the skin or splash to the eyes, but sometimes skin cuts could be small and unnoticed.

- Because the main transmission of HIV is by sexual contact through secretions, means to reduce direct contact with infected fluids is a priority. In the United States, there has always been an outcry for safe sex, which involves barrier precautions not only to prevent HIV transmission but also other sexually transmitted diseases. This concept is not embraced by many countries and cultures.

- The CDC launched a strategy for HIV prevention called the Serostatus Approach to Fighting the HIV Epidemic. This program is mostly about public health education. We also know that adherence to ART will reduce the viral load in blood and body secretions and statistically will reduce the risk of infection transmission.

- A number of special preventative strategies have been adopted for other cultures. While not acceptable for all cultures, male circumcision reduces the risk of HIV transmission. Testing of sexual partners to see if there is sero-discordance, with one partner HIV positive and the other HIV negative, could be important to prevent HIV transmission, although many do not get tested.

- The CDC and World Health Organization have recommended a strategy known as preexposure prophylaxis for those who are at high risk of acquiring HIV, including sero-discordant couples, couples not using condoms, and injection-drug users who share needles. This means the noninfected partner takes a limited ART regimen daily, not just before a high-risk encounter. When medications are reliably taken, the risk reduction may be as high as 90 percent.

- Control of HIV nationally and worldwide also requires extensive financial support. The United States has a plan called the President's Emergency Plan for AIDS Relief (PEPFAR), which is a program that targets resource-poor countries that are hit hardest by the HIV pandemic and is mostly coordinated by the CDC. In 2011, President Obama announced a vision of an AIDS-free generation via PEPFAR, which is committed to supporting 6 million AIDS patients who are in treatment and providing drug therapy for life to 1.5 million pregnant women and their babies.

Vaccine Development and Genetic Engineering

- In spite of all the prevention efforts, a vaccine will be required to end the global HIV pandemic. The challenge in the development of such a vaccine appears unprecedented. A vaccine that is modeled using classic vaccination concepts remains the ultimate goal for HIV. The vaccine would induce an immune response that prevents the establishment of HIV infection.

- The development of a vaccine that would produce broadly neutralizing antibodies, which could potentially halt primary infection, is a priority. The exact antigenic protein, or combination of proteins, to target for these antibodies has been elusive so far. We do know, however, that broadly neutralizing antibodies are produced in HIV-infected individuals, but unfortunately not for several years. We are not sure yet how to speed up this process.

- Also, in contrast to the relative ease of producing influenza vaccines, the genetic diversity and mutational capacity of HIV is much greater than that of influenza. This creates a larger challenge to attaining a vaccine. Because HIV rapidly integrates into the CD4 genome and establishes latent reservoirs of virus, any vaccine would also need to produce other T-helper lymphocytes that would control these latent sites.

- This goal may not be achievable with the first vaccination attempts. Instead, the first vaccine may need to be designed to reduce HIV viral levels and preserve uninfected CD4 cells. The natural history of HIV infection shows that the viral blood burden correlates with disease progression. Reducing viral RNA by one or more logarithms should slow disease progression.

- With all these frustrations facing researchers, some have turned their focus to a different strategy: modifying the genes of host CD4 cells to make them resistant to infection. It is also known that a small percent of humans lack a receptor on their CD4 cells, CCR5, and are immune to HIV. Conceptually, researchers are targeting the

CCR5 gene in stem cells to make the CD4 cells automatically lack the CCR5 receptor and naturally block infection.

Suggested Reading

Shilts, *And the Band Played On*.

Questions to Consider

1. Where did HIV virus come from, and why is it still so widespread worldwide?

2. Can you get HIV virus from casual contact, such as a kiss or a visit to the public restroom? If a friend of yours were infected, would you feel comfortable having him or her over for dinner?

Malaria and Tuberculosis: Global Killers

Lecture 19

In this lecture, you will learn about the two deadliest diseases in the world: malaria and tuberculosis (TB). In spite of a multitude of global efforts to decrease their mortality rates, these two devastating diseases affect a huge portion of the world's population. Malaria still manages to infect one out of every 21 human beings on the planet—300 million people yearly—and kills nearly 1 million humans year after year. One-third of the world's population has been exposed to TB, and in a recent year in the United States, there were still around 10,000 cases of TB.

Malaria

- In the 1890s, while studying malaria in India, British physician Ronald Ross discovered that mosquitoes were the transmitters of the disease. This, and other malaria research, eventually earned him the 1902 Nobel Prize in Medicine.

- The *Anopheles* species of mosquito is the only one of hundreds of mosquito species that carries the malaria parasite—known as *Plasmodia*. Only the female is responsible for malaria transmission. There are five species of plasmodia parasites that affect humans. The most virulent is *Plasmodia falciparum*, which causes 50 percent of infections and 95 percent of deaths. *Plasmodia* are so specialized at survival that they have both sexual and asexual forms of reproduction.

- Female mosquitoes bite us because they need the proteins from our blood in order to develop their eggs. Their saliva contains proteins that are transferred into humans as they feed. The proteins provoke an immune response in the form of local inflammation—a mosquito bite.

- When female mosquitoes feed on the blood of an infected human, it absorbs gametocytes, the sexual elements of the parasite—the equivalent to sperm or eggs. The gametocytes combine to form oocytes that burrow into the mosquito stomach. Growth and division of each oocyte produces thousands of active malaria forms called sporozoites. After a week or two, the oocyte bursts, releasing sporozoites that invade the mosquito salivary glands. The next time the mosquito bites, it releases these sporozoites from its salivary glands into the new human host.

- Next, the parasites move through the bloodstream directly to the liver, where they establish a parasitic state, taking over liver cells and replicating thousands of times. But their ultimate destination is not the liver. They break out of the liver cells and attach to—and then invade—the red blood cells of the circulatory system.

- The malaria parasites are resilient and also multiply further by taking over red blood cells and using sexual reproduction to proliferate even further. The immune system is triggered, causing a resetting of the body's thermostat. This causes fever to destroy the invaders, but even though it kills some, most remain. The surviving parasites take over the red blood cells, feeding on the hemoglobin as a nutrient source and continuing reproduction. The red blood cell counts fall, and there is not as much capacity to transport oxygen, which produces fatigue and weakness.

- At this point, what happens to the individual human is dependent on the species of parasite causing the infection. If the species is *Plasmodium vivax* or *ovale*, they cause milder symptoms and return to the liver. Approximately 72 hours later, they usually produce another wave of parasites to invade the blood. Usually, there are two or three waves of blood invasion before they settle into a hibernating state in the liver and spleen. They can remain in the liver to enter the blood weeks, months, or occasionally years later.

- This 72-hour time cycle is important because victims feel remarkably well in the 2 days between the 3-day parasite cycle. The fever pattern is actually a major clue to the diagnosis of malaria.

Each time the parasites are released into the blood, there is a loss of oxygen-carrying red blood cells. The liver and spleen also enlarge, because these organs act like large lymph nodes, trapping red-cell-laden parasites.

- One of the reasons malaria has survived as a parasitic disease for thousands of years is that *P. ovale* and *vivax* usually do not kill the human host. Instead, they act as a reservoir for transmission to others.

- The deadliest malaria species is *Falciparum*. During the blood stage, the *Falciparum* species has the ability to alter the red blood cells' surfaces, causing them to stick to blood vessel walls. This causes sludging of red cells and impairment of oxygen exchange to the brain.

- If untreated, the brain begins to swell, and malaria has reached its most deadly phase. By this time, so many red cells have been destroyed that the vital functions of the heart and lungs start failing, and the immune system is overwhelmed. Often, this scenario usually results in a coma, and then death.

- A treatment for malaria was discovered in Peru in the 1600s. It came from the bark of the cinchona tree, and it is still used as an inexpensive cure in some parts of the world. It is known as quinine. Later, this ingredient was chemically modified into chloroquine, the first synthetic antimalarial medication.

- All malaria used to be sensitive to chloroquine. However, malaria adapted to chloroquine and developed resistance over the course of a few decades. Now there are only a limited number of geographic locations in the world (the Caribbean and Latin America) where chloroquine is still effective.

- Other malaria medications are available and are mainly targeted toward the prevention of *Falciparum* malaria, because it's the deadliest. These include weekly treatments with mefloquine or daily Malarone or doxycycline.

- When traveling to endemic areas, it is recommended that you take preventive malaria medication. Malaria is still prevalent in 106 countries. There are ongoing efforts today by the World Health Organization to try to prevent and reduce malaria by the distribution of treated mosquito netting, educational efforts for the native population, aggressive medication treatments, and the spraying of insecticides to reduce the mosquito population. But this is not enough.

- The Bill & Melinda Gates Foundation has spent more than a billion dollars in an effort to eradicate malaria. They believe that the means to success will be by total eradication of the mosquito. This means that it is essential to use new technologies to develop and deliver a sustainable response to the mosquito population.

- One effort involves genetically modifying the male mosquito and its ability to transmit the X chromosome. Female species need two X chromosomes. At the Imperial College of London, scientists are injecting a biologically engineered gene into the male mosquito. This wipes out the X chromosome's DNA. Thereafter, males can only donate the Y chromosome, consequently reducing female populations.

- Another technique using genetically engineered sterile mosquitoes in the Cayman Islands wiped out 80 percent of the mosquito population there in 2010. As always, there are caveats to bioengineering: If you wipe out one species of mosquito, will another species' population rise? What effect will changing a region's ecosystem have over the long term? Time will tell.

- There is also hope with trials of an RTSS vaccine that contains part of a sporozoite protein. This is the stage of malaria that is inoculated by the feeding mosquito at the first moments of infection—before malaria gets to the liver. Trials resulted in a 50 percent reduction in malaria in African children. This *Falciparum* malaria vaccine hopefully will substantially reduce malaria in African children. Development of vaccines, and the eradication of mosquitoes, will continue to be two important efforts to prevent deaths from malaria.

Tuberculosis

- Worldwide, one person is infected with *Mycobacterium tuberculosis* every second. Robert Koch identified the TB germ in 1882 and named it "Koch's bacillus." In 1905, he won the Nobel Prize for his discovery. In early 1895, the X-ray was invented, which helped confirm diagnoses by provided images of TB disease in the chest.

- Why is it that TB has been around for thousands of years, and why is the incidence of infection so high? The main reason relates to the highly contagious potential of the bacteria: The size of the TB germ is about three microns in size, which is the same size as dust particles in the air. So, when someone with active TB coughs, he or she generates an aerosol of germs that does not sink to the ground

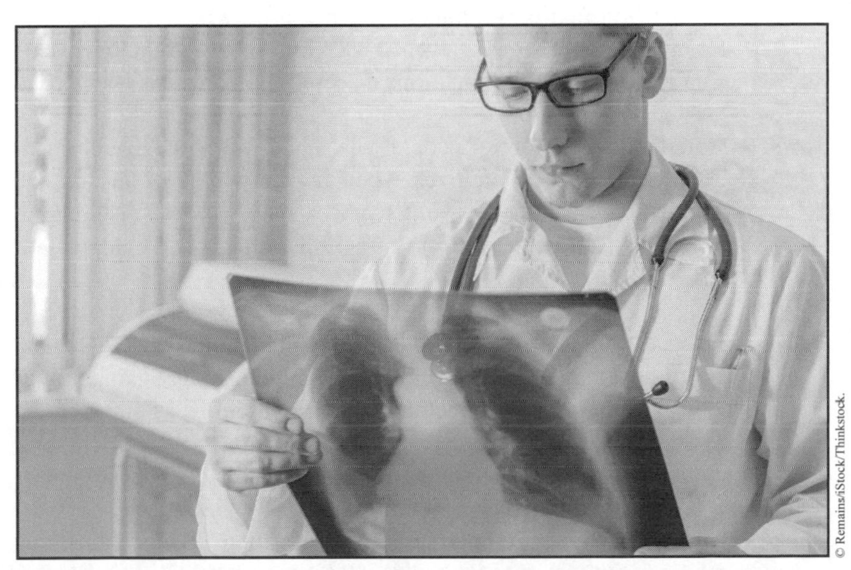

The invention of the X-ray helped to confirm diagnoses of tuberculosis in patients' chests.

in the six- to eight-foot radius like normal, larger germs. TB germs ride the air currents and can be spread over large distances.

- When individuals are exposed to air currents with TB, there is a high probability that TB will enter the lungs and settle in the furthest passages of the airways. This exposure begins a complex immune response by several different types of cells to attempt to contain TB to the lung.

- The germ is *Mycobacterium*, which differentiates itself from normal bacteria with a special outer membrane made of mycolic acid. This makes it more difficult for our immune system to contain and kill the germ. TB can continue to live inside of cells.

- Primary initial TB active infection from germ inhalation is prone to happen if there is a large number of TB germs inhaled at the start, if your immune system is compromised, or if you have the HIV virus. Under most circumstances, active TB does not immediately occur. But the best that our immune system can provide is to "wall off" TB in a highly organized layer of cells known as a granuloma. This usually leads to a noncontagious disease state known as latent TB.

- More than 90 percent of people who inhale TB will carry dormant TB bacteria their whole lives. Their bodies will show an immune response with antibodies and reactive lymphocytes, resulting in a positive TB skin test. Up to one-third of the world's population carries TB in a latent form.

- Especially in the first three years after inhalation, there is still a risk of developing active TB until the immune system gains further control of the original infection. More importantly, as our immune system ages, a small percentage of those with latent TB will lose containment of the TB that has been inactive for even decades.

- This leads to a condition known as reactivation TB. To reduce this risk with aging, patients with latent TB are usually offered a chance to take a single TB medication, called isoniazid, to reduce the risk of reactivation TB.

- Inside the bodies of people that develop active TB or reactivation TB, the bacteria leave the lungs, enter the bloodstream, and can settle anywhere in the body as disseminated, or miliary, TB. In most patients, the germ also returns to the lung, combining with the site of the original infection, leading to active lung TB. With a large burden of TB in the lung, the lung architecture can be destroyed, leading to cavitary TB—a hole in the lung.

- Over the past 30 years, because a large percentage of the African continent is infected with HIV, there has been a resurgence of TB as a major worldwide disease—the result of devastation to the immune system. It is estimated that more than 11 million people are infected with both TB and HIV. In the United States, it's estimated that up to 20 percent of patients with active TB are also HIV positive.

- TB usually requires treatment with four medications to start with, because each medication has a specific target in the layers within the granulomas surrounding the TB germs. The drugs are usually isoniazid, rifampin, pyrazinamide, and ethambutol.

- People who do not follow through with taking TB medications completely usually don't get well, and they increase the chances of developing drug-resistant TB. Or, by taking medications in a haphazard fashion, low concentrations of drugs will give the multiplying germs a chance at genetic mutations that will favor the emergence of resistant strains.

- For the first time in 40 years, though, the FDA has approved a new agent to treat drug-resistant TB, known as bedaquiline. There are several other new drugs under development with support from the Gates Foundation and others.

- Rather than containing and treating TB, prevention efforts with vaccination should be a priority—just like with malaria. There is a vaccine called bacillus Calmette–Guérin that is used in many countries outside the United States for vaccinating small children. This vaccine is a weakened form of a cow strain of TB. Its protective effect may reduce the risk of TB active disease by about 50 percent.

Suggested Reading

Ryan, *The Forgotten Plague*.

Shah, *The Fever*.

Waksman, *The Conquest of Tuberculosis*.

Questions to Consider

1. Why are so many children still dying every minute from malaria? What kind of precautions would you need to take if you traveled to parts of the world that have malaria?

2. What is it about the tuberculosis germ that continues to make it such a worldwide cause of death? How likely are you to catch tuberculosis in the United States?

Global Travel, War, and Natural Disasters

Lecture 20

This lecture continues to address global infectious disease issues and the toll they take on populations. Specifically, you will learn about the public health effects of wars and natural disasters. You also will explore the health risks associated with worldwide travel and the precautions you need to take to stay healthy. In addition, you will learn about the systems and organizations that are tasked with monitoring health in the Unites States and all over the world.

Syria's Civil War

- In November of 2013, the World Health Organization (WHO) confirmed a polio outbreak in Syria, which had been free of polio since 1999. However, since war broke out in 2011, the polio immunization rate fell from 91 percent to 33 percent. That meant that around half of a million children were vulnerable to polio. The public health system has disintegrated, with over half of their medical facilities damaged, and there is a shortage of precious antibiotics and vaccines.

- A typhoid epidemic, caused by salmonella bacteria, also erupted. In addition to polio, viral hepatitis, measles, and mumps surfaced—thought to have originated from the influx of unvaccinated Pakistani fighters into Syria.

- Syria itself is already hosting more than 100,000 refugees from other war-torn countries, including Iraq, Afghanistan, and Somalia. There were over 4 million displaced citizens in Syria who were in need of aid. Damage to roads and infrastructure complicated health-care efforts to reach remote areas. A massive immunization effort was undertaken targeting the refugees and native parts of Syria that could still be reached by aid workers.

- Contagious diseases were spreading by the fecal-oral route due to contaminated water from rivers and wells. The increasingly large piles of garbage were causing more sand flies to swarm, transmitting an ulcerous parasitic skin infection called leishmaniasis. The situation appeared unmanageable, and the outlook was dim.

- In nearby countries, almost 2 million Syrian refugees took shelter in camps or host communities. These conditions in refugee camps involved inadequate clean water, lack of food, lack of sanitation, and limited access to medical care. Refugee camps on the Turkish-Syrian border began to experience cases of cholera and malaria.

- Because Turkey shares an 850-kilometer border with Syria, it was impossible to monitor and register all refugees crossing the border. Some Syrians crossing the border are sick and will bring new diseases to areas where they were not prevalent. They may continue to make their way across Turkey and into Europe, creating a further potential for disease spread.

- Host countries are bulging at the seams, dealing with increasing health threats to their own populations. In addition, their own resources are being diverted to the overwhelming numbers of refugees pouring in. This formula yields the perfect breeding ground for infectious diseases to spread at a rapid pace to contiguous countries. Wherever there is war, this health-care disaster scenario will continue to occur with similar themes.

Natural Disasters

- War is a manmade disaster, but natural disasters can have equally devastating effects on human health. The first thought on most people's minds is that the post-disaster environment becomes a breeding ground for disease. But, as a general rule, the risk for outbreaks from the natural disaster itself is low; the risks actually result from displaced populations. People are forced to live in conditions that are crowded, with a lack of sanitation and clean water, and a lack of medical access.

- There was a cholera epidemic that occurred in Haiti after the earthquake in 2010. The cholera strain that killed thousands of Haitians was likely brought into Haiti by a UN Nepalese disaster response team. There was an active cholera outbreak in Nepal at the time the soldiers were transferred to Haiti, and the soldiers were not tested for cholera before leaving their posts in Nepal.

- The disease broke out several months after the peacekeepers' arrival. They lived on a base with inadequate sanitation, so fecal matter entered the rivers. The rivers' water was used for bathing, drinking, washing, and recreation. All of the victims in the early stages of the outbreak had consumed water from this river.

- So, cholera had nothing to do with the earthquake. This event infected 700,000 and resulted in more than 8,500 deaths. Prevention and close monitoring of the early outbreak could have prevented thousands of deaths that yielded a double dose of misery in Haiti.

- Oral and intravenous hydration fluids, as well as the antibiotic doxycycline, can save many lives if the supplies are available. The WHO controls three licensed formulations of cholera vaccine for worldwide outbreaks. Vaccine efficacy ranges from 66 to 85 percent. Unfortunately, the WHO did not initiate vaccine efforts in Haiti until late in the outbreak.

- Victims of the tornado in Joplin, Missouri, in 2011 suffered from mucormycosis, a rare but serious fungal infection that can start as a skin infection but disseminate throughout the body and become deadly. This happened because flying debris, containing soil contaminated with the fungus mucor, penetrated the skin and infected wounds.

- In the 1800s, in addition to malaria, New Orleans suffered outbreaks of cholera and typhoid fever, because contaminated water was hospitable for breeding germs in the most tropical environment in the United States. Over time, an improved public health system kept epidemics at bay. But after Hurricane Katrina in 2010, several infectious diseases became problematic again.

- Whenever there is raw sewage in the streets, or standing water, there is potential for disease. This could include bacteria from animal and human feces, as well as rotting biological matter. For example, hepatitis A virus is spread from contaminated food or water, so this is an issue with all flooding, because adults are not normally vaccinated against it. In addition, standing water from flooding increases the mosquito population and increases the potential spreading of new diseases, such as West Nile virus.

Global Travel Precautions

- With the number of international travelers rising each year, particularly traveling to developing countries, how do you know if it's medically safe to travel to certain areas? Interestingly, demand for international tourism in 2013 was strongest for travel to countries with the most infectious disease potential: Southeast Asia, Eastern Europe, and North Africa. This means that people need to ideally prepare themselves for health risks months in advance and must monitor the situation in these areas on a regular basis.

- The U.S. State Department posts travelers' safety and health warnings; however, they are not the only organization that is constantly monitoring outbreaks and epidemics around the world. For example, in 2014, the Centers for Disease Control and Prevention (CDC) posted warnings for 10 countries for polio on their website. It also posts occurrences of natural disasters and the potential health implications for travelers.

- The CDC's travel site allows you to plug in information relevant to your trip and will give you information about associated infectious disease health risks. Having this information allows you time to get the needed vaccines and to pack both insect repellent and insect-repellent clothing.

- You can also receive helpful recommendations for water precautions, such as taking a water bottle and water-purifying tablets along, or buying a water bottle that has a special filter. For example, the LIFESAVER bottle claims to remove all bacteria, viruses, cysts, parasites, fungi, and waterborne pathogens—even poliovirus and *E. coli*.

- There is a wise saying that when you eat food in developing countries, you should either peel it, boil it, cook it, or forget it. For example, don't eat foods like salads, raw fruits and vegetables, raw or runny eggs, food at room temperature, or so-called bushmeat. For drinks, realize that ice cubes are often contaminated, so stick to bottled drinks and pasteurized beverages. Under most circumstances, you should even brush your teeth with bottled water, just to be safe.

- The CDC website is a valuable place to start, but travel clinics have special resources as well. Travel clinics are especially important if you're going to an area of either South America or Africa where yellow fever is endemic. Yellow fever is caused by a potentially deadly virus that is mosquito-borne, rapidly attacks the liver, and leads to yellow jaundice. Only certified travel clinics can administer the yellow fever vaccine, and an official booklet stamp is required to enter other countries after visiting countries with yellow fever risk.

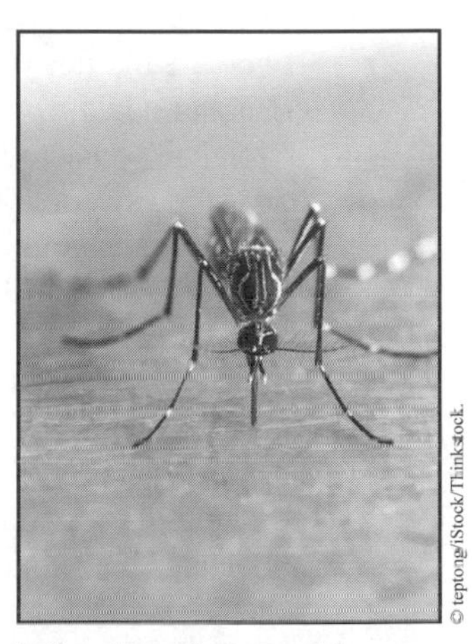

Yellow fever is caused by a mosquito-borne virus that is endemic in some areas of South America and Africa.

- Some vaccines need multiple injections and have to be given in a series, months apart. This means that you have to work backward in your timetable in order to be fully protected by the time of your trip.

Health officials recommend finishing all vaccines at least one week before traveling, in case you have any rare side effects and in order to give your immune system time to form antibodies. Additional planning is also important so that you can identify medical care availability in the area where you are traveling.

- If you buy traveler's health insurance, they usually work with specific providers in the countries they serve. Otherwise, there is a list of organizations you can contact in case of emergencies, such as the U.S. embassy and the International Association for Medical Assistance to Travellers.

- If you are ill after your trip, hopefully you kept track of places you went and noted if you were bitten by any insects during that time, if you had contact with animals, what kind of food and drinks you had, if you swam in lakes or rivers, etc. These are important pieces of information your doctor will need to know to create a differential diagnosis for your illness.

Public Health Surveillance

- During wartime or during natural disasters or outbreaks, public health surveillance is critical to providing evidence for sound decision making during crises. It provides a formal system of collecting, analyzing, interpreting, and disseminating data.

- The WHO monitors trends, disseminates information, and hosts the Global Health Observatory. This is a data repository for health-related topics, such as world health statistics, specific disease statistics, and environmental risks with formal reports.

- Data from informal sources, such as telephone calls from individuals reporting urgent health events all over the world, are welcome. Suspicious informal reporting allows for a potentially earlier response to health threats.

- The GeoSentinel Surveillance Network has been monitoring health around the world for more than a decade. This network has 57 medical clinics throughout each continent that continually collect information on ill travelers, immigrants, or refugees who have gone to these clinics. The clinics fax information to a central data site, where it is aggregated. In this way, unusual illnesses in unusual locations are quickly communicated to partners to assess trends in populations and areas and to share information.

- Both the CDC's National Center for Emerging and Zoonotic Infectious Diseases and the International Society for Infectious Diseases are heavily involved in preventing diseases and deaths due to infectious diseases, using the One Health strategy. They also publish the current outbreak list and ProMED digest, which lists all domestic and foreign infectious disease events and outbreaks.

- The Animal and Plant Health Inspection Service coordinates efforts to monitor plants and animals coming into the United States to ensure that they do not carry any diseases that can be transmitted.

- Social media has helped in various disaster situations. Videos are taken by bystanders who bear witness to the devastating circumstances of war and post them on YouTube for the world to see. For example, using YouTube videos that provided real-time information in Syria, clinicians were able to firmly conclude that sarin nerve gas had been used, based on the signs affecting the victims.

- Pictures are sent on TwitPic to show the reality of desperate situations; in fact, donations to the Red Cross for Haiti relief poured in over text messages pledging 10 dollars each, adding up to more than 30 million dollars. Also, after Haiti's earthquake in 2010, Ushahidi—an open-source web platform—used information that was crowd-sourced to link health-care providers who needed supplies to the people who had the supplies.

- The One Health Initiative is a collaborative effort among human, animal, and environmental health professionals. It is important to collaborate and share information about all three elements to identify potential dangers and to coordinate response efforts. Many of the emerging infectious diseases are zoonotic, and many emerge because of destruction of the environment. We are inextricably linked to the health of all three of these facets of life.

Suggested Reading

Atlas and Maloy, *One Health*.

Zinsser, *Rats, Lice and History*.

Questions to Consider

1. If you are planning a trip overseas, what preventative measures would you take in advance to avoid getting sick? Once you are there, how can you stay well?

2. What technology would you use on an international trip in order to keep apprised of outbreaks?

Influenza: Past and Future Threat

Lecture 21

You might think of the flu season as just a regular annual occurrence: If you catch it, you have a 7- to 10-day bout of misery and then return to work. But you might not know that there have been four full-fledged worldwide influenza outbreaks—some of the deadliest pandemics of all time. In this lecture, you will learn about the influenza virus and how it causes human disease. In addition, you will learn what makes influenza stand out from other respiratory illnesses and how influenza is prevented with vaccination.

Influenza Types

- Seasonal flus are caused by influenza types A and B. Influenza A can infect both humans and animals. It has the highest pandemic potential due to the possibility for mixing animal and human RNA, leading to surface protein mutations. Influenza B is a human virus only, has much less mutational capacity than type A, and has only one set of surface proteins—and, hence, is one species. But there are slight structural variations of flu B that give influenza B strain numbers instead. Strains are determined by the city and year where it originated, such as B/Shanghai361/2002.

- Influenza C is a human flu that causes very mild respiratory illness and often is not even recognized as causing classic clinical influenza illness. Importantly, neither flu B nor C is associated with pandemics, meaning that there is global spread of a disease. Alternatively, influenza in the United States on a yearly basis is an epidemic, meaning that the disease rapidly spreads to many people in a limited geographic region.

- Influenza virus is an RNA virus in the *Orthomyxovirus* family. Like all viruses, it can't replicate by itself. It needs to take over the protein machinery of a living cell and reprogram the cell to create more viral particles, which usually results in cell death.

- Type A virus is covered on its envelope, or outside surface, with two types of foreign protein spikes known by the letters "H" and "N." "H" is an abbreviation of the word "hemagglutinin," and "N" is an abbreviation for "neuraminidase."

- The H spike is used like a hook by the virus to attach itself to the outside of a host cell. The cytoplasmic membrane of the cell then engulfs the virus and pulls it inside. Through a complicated series of maneuvers—including uncoating of the virus, where the RNA slips out of its viral coating—the virus tricks the host cell to let the viral RNA into the cell interior. Once this occurs, the virus is in control. Remarkably, within about 12 hours of hijacking the cell, the influenza virus can release up to one million new viruses. With such a rapid rate, there is a high possibility for genetic mutations.

- The antiviral medications amantadine and rimantadine were effective against the influenza A virus for many years. Both medications inhibited virus replication by interfering with the viral uncoating process heading inside the cell. Importantly, the high mutation rate of influenza A has led to the emergence of widespread resistance to both these antiviral medications, and neither is used for treatment anymore.

- The N spike is essential for the virus to break out of its host cell, essentially performing the opposite of the H spike, cutting holes in the cell membrane from the inside to allow the viruses to escape and infect other cells.

- Antiviral medications known as neuraminidase inhibitors are fortunately still effective at shutting down virus replication. Oseltamivir and zanamivir are two of these antiviral medications. They work against both influenza A and B, and so far viruses have shown a very low mutation rate against them. The antiviral medications inhibit the release of the virus from the host cell by blocking neuraminidase—so, basically, it can't replicate.

- When these antiviral medications are given within the first 72 hours of influenza illness, they can shorten the duration of clinical illness by one or two days. They have also been shown to reduce the rate of secondary bacterial infections of the lung.

- Antiviral medications are deemed to be helpful in those unfortunate enough to be hospitalized for influenza, even when the 72-hour window has expired. In general, the earlier they are given, the more clinical benefit antiviral medications are likely to have. They can also judiciously be used for prophylaxis, or prevention, of flu when there are outbreak circumstances in a closed institution, such as a nursing home.

Nomenclature

- Why is a virus called H1N1? The virus has hemagglutinin type 1 protein (for the H1 protein) and neuraminidase type 1 protein (for the N1 protein). There are 16 versions of hemagglutinin and 9 versions of neuraminidasc, so you can expect to see many combinations of influenza A viruses in the future.

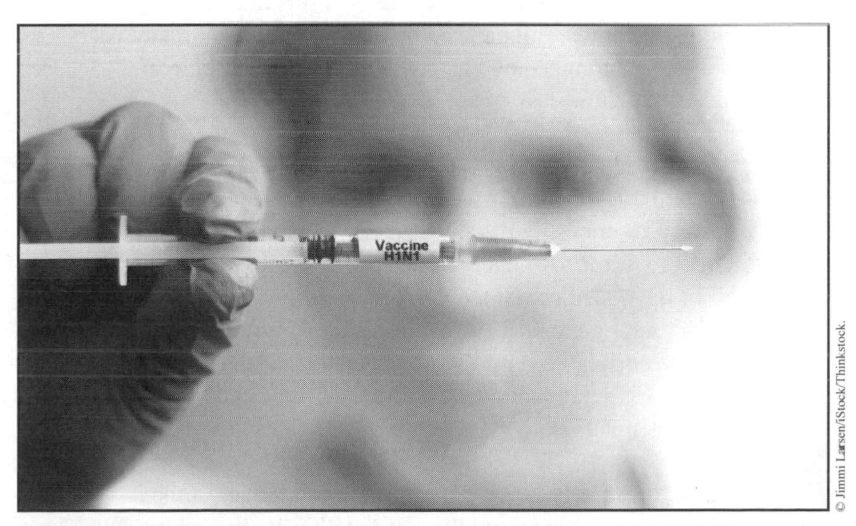

H1N1, also known as "swine flu," is a type of virus that is named for the certain proteins it contains.

- Antigenic drift, a process in which mutations to the virus genome produce changes in the viral H or N proteins, results in the emergence of new strains when either the H or the N protein undergoes minor changes—H1N1 to H1N2 or to H2N1.

- This is why the flu vaccine contains a different mix of viruses each year and must be updated annually. Because this is a single mutation, however, usually our bodies recognize at least one of the two proteins. We still experience a partial immune response that helps us fight the virus.

- Antigenic shift, on the other hand, is the reason that pandemic viruses arise. Instead of modifying the existing H and N proteins, the proteins are replaced by significantly different Hs and Ns—for example, H1N1 to H5N2. This means that our bodies do not recognize either of these new Hs and Ns, and therefore we do not have any preexisting antibody protection against them.

- A pandemic is usually caused by a new strain of virus or a reappearing old one. These are viruses that either have never circulated among humans before or that circulated many years ago. So, either humans have no immunity against it or very little. This makes the virus easy to spread.

- Since 1918—when an epidemic of influenza designated as an H1N1, or "swine flu," variety left Spain's population growth rate in negative numbers—all influenza-A pandemics have been caused by viruses with RNA genetic remnants of the 1918 virus. In addition, all of them also contained RNA from swine. However, importantly, the internal genetic RNA composition of influenza viruses is only loosely correlated with the nomenclature of the H and N proteins. So, the 1918 pandemic earned the right to be called the "mother" of all pandemics.

- So far, there have been four influenza pandemics in the last century, which spread throughout the world within six to nine months. These pandemics were the 1918 Spanish flu, the 1957 Asian flu, the 1968

Hong Kong flu, and the 2009 Mexican flu. Because the speed and frequency of air travel has significantly increased since the 1960s, a much faster spread of influenza was seen in the 2009 pandemic.

- Pandemic viruses can also occur when some of the genes from animal flu viruses mix with genes from human flu viruses to create a new hybrid. This happens when an animal or person is coinfected by both a human virus and an avian flu virus at the same time. The process of combining viruses is called reassortment. In fact, the 2009 swine flu virus was a combination of swine, bird, and human flu viruses.

- It's difficult to believe that the descendants of the 1918 virus still persist in pigs today. After the 1957 Asian flu, the H1N1 descendants of the 1918 strain had seemingly disappeared from human circulation, until human H1N1 viruses suddenly reappeared in 1977.

- The 1977 swine flu first emerged at Fort Dix, NJ, and killed several soldiers. This was the impetus for the urgent creation of a swine flu vaccine that 40 million U.S. citizens received in record time. This vaccination effort was shrouded in controversy because it may have caused a slight increase in the incidence of a rare neurologic disorder, Guillain-Barré syndrome. Also, the pandemic never occurred.

- So, the side effects of vaccination overshadowed the positive aspects of rapid vaccine development and a mass public health response and made many people reluctant to get routine influenza vaccinations for years after the event.

Influenza-Like Illness

- The term "influenza-like illness" (ILI) is used to describe the influenza symptom complex. There is usually an incubation period of one to four days between the time the virus is acquired and illness begins. Not everyone with ILI has true influenza. In fact, there are many viruses that can mimic influenza, and several go by the strains of virus known as parainfluenza 1, 2, and 3. There are others.

- Usually, ILI begins with a runny nose and upper respiratory congestion for 24 hours, while the virus is gaining entry into the surface cells lining the nose and mucous membranes of the head. In the next 24 hours, sore throat and headache symptoms begin.

- The headache of true influenza seems to be relatively distinctive compared with other ILI, usually toward the front of the head and with the distinction that moving your eyes back and forth elicits discomfort in your eye sockets.

- Usually, fever begins during the second day. But this is just the beginning. Within the next 24 hours, the virus invades the bloodstream, breaking through the respiratory linings. True influenza virus has a propensity to invade muscles, sometimes leading to agonizing muscle aches and a feeling of inability to move. The virus also descends into the upper airways of the lung, usually causing a dry, nonproductive cough with white phlegm.

- In order to fight the viral infection, the body starts to mount a higher fever—trying to kill the virus—of usually 102 to 103 degrees. The resetting of the body's thermostat often leads to episodes of shaking chills that at times may feel uncontrollable.

- Even three days into the illness, relief does not come quickly. The main symptoms persist for up to another 72 hours, before finally scaling down on the seventh day of the illness. It may still take days to get back to feeling normal. While most people will recover, presently influenza leads to the hospitalization of more than 200,000 people yearly and results in 30,000 to 50,000 deaths from flu or flu-related complications in the United States.

Vaccination

- There has been an advance in the flu vaccine, moving from two flavors of type A strains and one flavor of type B to a vaccine with two strains of both A and B. We call this a quadrivalent vaccine, and it has more opportunity for successful protection. Other changes to prior vaccination policy include allowing most patients with egg allergies to still be vaccinated; recommending that children ages two to eight receive the live, rather than killed, flu vaccine; and preferring a high-dose vaccine for those over the age of 65, for better prevention efficacy.

- Because the manufacturing of the vaccine takes several months, how does the World Health Organization determine which strains of influenza will be targeted in the vaccine for the fall? This is an important decision, one that involves influenza experts from all over the world. If the wrong strain is chosen for production, the efficacy of the vaccine will be more limited.

- In general, the Northern Hemisphere takes its clue for vaccine composition from the Southern Hemisphere, and vice versa, because the seasons are reversed. In February, they decide on the vaccine for the next Northern Hemisphere season based on information gathered from influenza centers in 100 countries and other partners that conduct global surveillance year-round.

- The exact reason for the seasonality of most strains of influenza in temperate climates has been studied in detail but is not definitively known. Influenza exists at a low level throughout the year but exhibits a marked seasonal increase during the winter months.

- It is probably a combination of factors, including cooler temperatures and lower humidity, which favor virus survival outside humans. Also, more crowded indoor environments in the winter play a role in this increase. Influenza occurs in tropical areas as well, but not typically with the same seasonality.

- In the future, scientists conceptually believe that history will repeat itself and that it is not a matter of whether there will be another influenza pandemic but a matter of when it will be and with which strain of the virus. Proactive plans are in place should this horrible event ever occur.

Suggested Reading

Barry, *The Great Influenza*.

Byerly, *Fever of War*.

Crosby, *America's Forgotten Pandemic*.

Questions to Consider

1. Why is there such a fuss about influenza illness and prevention every year? Why is there a different vaccination every year?

2. What lessons does the great influenza pandemic of 1918 have to teach us about the future of infectious diseases?

Bioterrorism: How Worried Should We Be?

Lecture 22

This lecture is about bioterrorism, which is the intentional release of viruses, bacteria, or other germs that have the potential to devastate our food supply, infest the water, contaminate the air, and ultimately sicken or kill people. Experts say that bioterrorism will happen—it's not a "maybe" anymore. In this lecture, you will explore the modern threat of bioterrorism and the agents that might be used in an attack. Specifically, you will learn how anthrax and botulism cause illness and how they can be treated.

Bioweapons

- There have been efforts in the 20th century to curtail the use of bioweapons. For example, in 1925, the Geneva Protocol was established, prohibiting the use of chemical and biological agents—but not the research and development of them. Today, we suspect that there are bioweapons in at least 12 countries, spurring the need for preparedness among medical and public health organizations.

- What is unique about planning a bioweapons attack as compared to others of mass destruction? For one thing, biological agents are likely to be smaller and more difficult to detect. They can be portable and easy to carry on different modes of transportation, and terrorists could disperse a bioweapons agent and leave the scene of the crime before anyone even showed symptoms of an illness. The acquisition expense is likely to be much cheaper as well.

- The Centers for Disease Control and Prevention places bioterrorist agents into three categories. These are based on the availability of the agent, its potential for infection or death, and how easily it could be disseminated. The most concerning agents are those in category A. These agents have characteristics that make them particularly worrisome.
    - They can be produced on a large scale.

- They can be aerosolized, making them easily transmittable.
- There is usually a lack of effective treatment or vaccines.
- Attacks could result in many casualties with a high mortality rate.

- The big six in category A include anthrax, smallpox, the plague, botulinum toxin, tularemia, and hemorrhagic viral fevers (such as Ebola). There are three scenarios that pose the greatest threats to us in a bioterrorism attack: an attack by an airborne agent (such as anthrax), a smallpox attack, and a release of botulinum toxin in cold drinks.

Anthrax

- Anthrax spores are easily found in nature or can be produced in a lab. It can be released in several forms, including in the form of powder, or spore forms could be aerosolized and released into the air and spread by the wind. It can be put into food and water, attacking people when they eat contaminated food or drink contaminated water.

- Inhalation anthrax is the most serious form of disease and would need immediate treatment for any chance at survival. It is odorless and invisible, and because the spores hitch a ride on dust particles in the air, they have been known to spread for up to 60 miles. A 1993 estimate predicted that 100 kilograms of aerosolized anthrax over a city would cause up to 3 million deaths—as lethal as a hydrogen bomb.

- Anthrax is an oxygen-loving, gram-positive, and spore-forming bacterium that lives in the soil and can contaminate wild animals. The anthrax bacterium looks like a bamboo rod with joints. Spores germinate when they find a welcoming host, such as the tissue or blood of animals or humans. It also may take only one to three spores to cause infection. If inhaled in the lung, the bacteria divide and produce a lethal toxin that can enter the circulation. This results in the sepsis syndrome.

- If anthrax is suspected to be in a patient's system, blood samples are taken and cultured in an incubator to enhance bacterial growth. If germs are detected in the blood, a gram stain can be done to look at the morphology of the bacteria. If they look like bamboo rods, the situation is highly suspicious for anthrax.

- Next, biochemical testing can be done to identify the specific bacteria. This usually takes another 12 to 24 hours. Usually, we initiate antibiotic treatment before the germ is completely identified—for example, after the gram stain is done on the blood—because the mortality consequences of waiting for confirmation could be dire.

- Anthrax is treatable with antibiotics, especially when recognized early. Today, we usually use ciprofloxacin, in part because it was rumored that the Russians had developed a penicillin-resistant form of anthrax for use as a bioweapon.

Botulism

- There are some very good reasons we worry about botulism toxin. By weight, it's the most poisonous substance known to man; 1 gram that is aerosolized has the potential to kill 1 million people. Like anthrax, the bacteria also germinate from spores. The *Clostridium* bacterium is easily obtained from soil, could be cultivated to produce toxin, and could be put into our food supply.

- Bacteria produce the toxin, which can enter the bloodstream from mucous membranes, the intestines, or cuts in the skin. The toxin will then bind to nerve endings. Normally, nerve conduction to activate muscle contraction depends on acetylcholine, a neurotransmitter.

- The botulism toxin blocks acetylcholine, which prevents muscles from contracting. Paralysis ensues, usually starting from the head and progressing downward toward the legs. When the disease is clinically recognized, the antidote is botulism antitoxin injected into the body.

- There are eight subtypes of botulism toxin, but the ones likely to be encountered in a bioterrorist attack are types A and B food-borne botulism—caused by eating foods that are contaminated with the toxin. Symptoms begin 12 to 72 hours after exposure with fatigue and dizziness, blurred vision, dry mouth, confusion, and then arm and leg weakness.

- Outside of a bioterrorist attack, an important health-care tip for parents and grandparents is that children under one year of age should not eat honey because it can contain the spores that can cause infant botulism. The spores are ingested and germinate in the child's large intestine, producing the neurotoxin. This leads to extreme muscle weakness, hence the term "floppy baby syndrome." The toxin can also attack the diaphragm, the muscle between the lungs and the stomach that controls respiration, causing suffocation. Infant botulism would be treated with an antitoxin.

- So, knowing that botulinum toxin is the most deadly substance known to mankind, why are people having it injected into their faces? Botox is one of four commercial products containing the type-A toxin, which is mixed with saline and injected into muscles. In fact, it is being used not only for cosmetic purposes, but for 20 other medical conditions.

- Why don't people die from injections of the toxin? The answer is that botulism poisoning is very dose-dependent. The lethal dose for a human is approximately 40 nanograms, where a nanogram is less than a millionth of a gram. The typical Botox injection for cosmetic purposes is about 8 nanograms.

- There are increasingly frequent cases of illegal sales of cloned Botox. This means that the toxin is getting purchased on the Internet and even from some manufacturers that don't require a prescription. It was even sold on eBay for a short time as a do-it-yourself kit.

- Scientists speculate that with a master's degree in biology and 2,000 dollars of equipment, an individual could hypothetically make enough toxin to kill thousands of people. So, we should be concerned about this scenario, especially in civilian populations that are unprepared. The only comforting news is that it seems to be poorly suited for delivery via bomb or missile, because it degrades quickly when exposed to heat.

Smallpox

- It's ironic that just when we think we've conquered smallpox, we have to fear that it still resides in labs around the world and could be used for bioterrorism. The United States government has obtained enough of the newest smallpox vaccine to treat 2 million people in the event of a bioterrorism attack. They even have a priority list of vaccine candidates, including health-care first responders, for example. The vaccine can prevent disease even if it is administered three days after exposure.

- Smallpox is feared for several reasons, including the lack of antiviral treatments, the fact that most people are not immune to the virus, and because it is highly contagious by aerosolized particles or contact with pox.

- The last few vials of smallpox are currently being held in high-security labs in the United States and Russia. Approximately every five years, the World Health Organization (WHO) meets to make an important decision: Should they eliminate the virus completely or save the remaining vials? Although destroying the vials would prevent the virus from being used as a terror-related weapon, leading virologists argue that the stock should be kept for research purposes, just in case the virus reemerges in the future.

- For the last 30 years, the WHO has not made the decision to fully destroy the remaining vials. In 2014, the almost unthinkable happened: Two vials of smallpox were found in a storage freezer box at the National Institutes of Health. The box seemed to date to the 1950s but had only been hiding in that location since 1972—obviously not where it was supposed to be. This, of course, resulted in protocols being reexamined and better security.

How to Know If We Are under a Bioterrorist Attack

- It is difficult to identify the early stages of a bioterrorist attack for several reasons. First, it is not until medical facilities begin to be overwhelmed with large numbers of victims with similar symptoms that epidemiologists begin to suspect either an epidemic or a bioterrorist attack. If the biological agent happens to be spread by human-to-human contact, it's likely that 10 to 12 other individuals would have already been infected. That makes it difficult to trace the source of the attack and try to contain it.

- What would be the first signs of a bioterrorist attack? There are some epidemiological clues you might see, including the following.
    - You might see an unusual illness pattern cropping up in the wrong season or in a non-endemic area. For example, it would be strange to see a large number of tularemia cases in a geographic area without the appropriate animal vectors.

    - You might also see an illness that is unusual for a particular population—for example, a large number of measles cases in adults.

    - You might even see a large number of animals dying, which would act as a sentinel event.

- Individual vigilance and health department surveillance are essential. In addition, the One Health Initiative is important, because clues could come from both animals and humans.

Preparedness for Any Type of Emergency

- Should you be preparing for a bioterrorist attack? The CDC's website has information on how to put together an emergency kit, how to develop a family disaster plan, and how to stay informed during an emergency of this type.

- Kits should contain similar supplies that you would need for natural disasters, such as tornadoes and hurricanes. Also think about including important personal documents. They would also include some specialized items, such as enhanced N95 masks, which would filter the air against TB, smallpox, and anthrax but would not help during a chemical or gas attack.

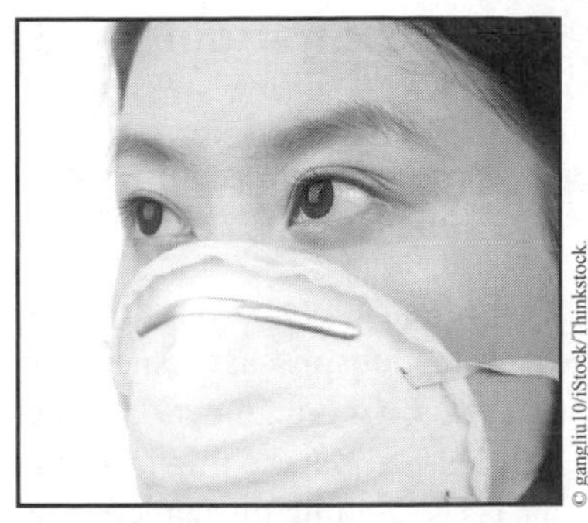
© gangliu10/iStock/Thinkstock.

N95 masks filter the air to help prevent the contraction of certain airborne diseases.

- One helpful medical advance that has been developed is the microbial detection array, which can detect more than 2,000 viruses and 900 types of bacteria within 24 hours. Its newer version will have double or triple this capacity. The array uses more than 380,000 probes, or nucleic acid sequences, which are microbe signatures. The probes fit on a l-by-3-inch glass slide. DNA or RNA samples are applied to the slide, read by a scanner, and analyzed using special algorithms. Rapid diagnostic testing capabilities will continue to be powerful tools not only in bioterrorist attacks, but in controlling disease outbreaks as well.

Suggested Reading

Cole, *Clouds of Secrecy*.

Mangold and Goldberg, *Plague Wars*.

Questions to Consider

1. Do we really have to be worried about bioterrorism in the United States? What would be the germ that might cause the most deaths?

2. What might be the first signs of a bioterrorism attack, and how can your family be prepared in advance if such an event actually happened?

Emerging and Reemerging Diseases

Lecture 23

In this lecture, you will learn about emerging, reemerging, and unknown infectious diseases, such as dengue, Ebola, MERS and SARS, West Nile virus, Chikungunya, measles, mumps, and pertussis. In addition, you will learn about the implications of these deadly diseases for all of us. These diseases continually challenge our detection and response abilities. There are no global boundaries with infectious diseases, so they should be a concern to all human beings all over the world.

Dengue

- The dengue virus is a leading cause of illness and sometimes death in the tropics. It has become important to people in the United States today because of its new environment in the Caribbean and even rare cases moving into the Florida Keys and Texas.

- The symptoms of dengue are high fever, severe headache, severe pain behind the eyes, and muscle and bone pain that last up to a week. A small proportion of dengue cases will progress to severe dengue, referred to as dengue hemorrhagic fever and dengue shock syndrome.

- Recent studies estimate that, worldwide, roughly 400 million dengue virus infections occur each year. About one-fourth of these infected individuals will have symptoms of the disease, and the remaining infections will be asymptomatic or subclinical. Because of overlapping symptoms, dengue is frequently misdiagnosed as malaria.

- As with other zoonotic diseases, the vector—the mosquito—is infected with dengue when it bites a person who has the virus in his or her blood. It then bites others, who become infected, resulting in a vicious cycle. It cannot be transmitted person to person, though.

- Current efforts are focusing on a dengue vaccine. Three of five vaccine candidates are of the live-attenuated type. Although current dengue vaccines do not offer complete protection against all four virus types, there were reductions of about 50 percent in dengue cases in clinical trials.

Ebola

- The outbreak of Ebola in 2014 in West Africa became an international crisis in a matter of weeks—involving contiguous West African countries at first, but hopping planes to the United States later. Beginning in Guinea, then spreading to Sierra Leone and Liberia, more than 10,000 cases were confirmed with a death rate of more than 50 percent.

- Viral hemorrhagic fevers have been around in West Africa for decades but have stayed within Africa until now. These are all RNA viruses, with Ebola part of the *Filovirus* family. Other virus

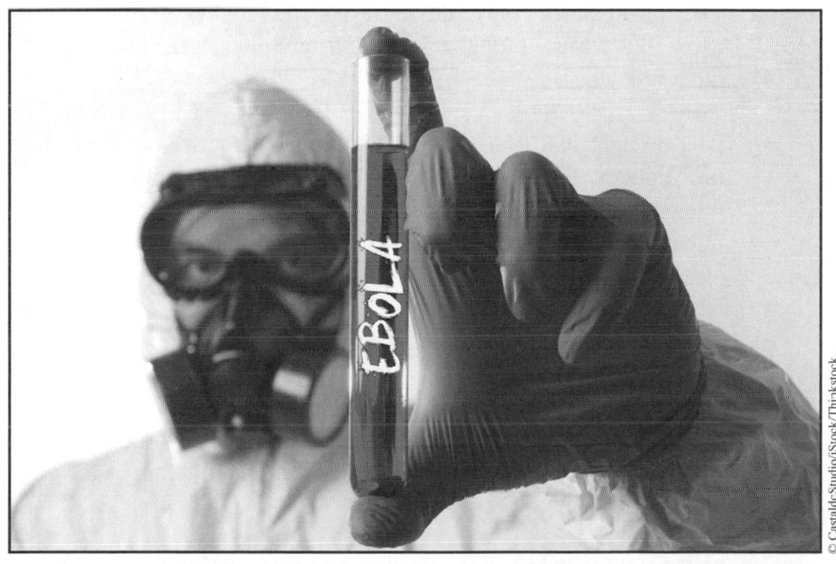

The Ebola virus is found in bodily fluids, so people caring for victims are at risk.

examples in the group include Lassa fever, Rift Valley fever, and Marburg virus. Infections cause victims to bleed uncontrollably in multiple organ systems, including intestinal fluid losses that can rival cholera. Without proper and immediate medical care, death will rapidly occur.

- There are five different types of Ebola virus, named after the places where they originated. Ebola has a characteristic shape of a stylized key. The outbreak was so significant that governments revived a disease-fighting measure that had not been used in nearly a century, known as cordon sanitaire. This means that an imaginary line is drawn around the infected area and no one is allowed to leave.

- Ebola was first discovered in 1976 in the Congo and is named after the Ebola River in that country. Scientists aren't exactly sure where the virus originated, but they think that fruit bats are the likely culprits. After bats were thought to be the host, Guinea implemented a ban on bat soup, which is a common street food. They also banned consumption of rats and monkeys. Other animals carry the virus, though, including chimpanzees, gorillas, and other monkeys.

- It is thought that transmission between countries is explained by the flight of bats. Scientists believe that the original method of transmission to humans was either directly from bats or by handling infected animals that were infected by bats.

- Because the virus is found in bodily fluids, such as human blood, urine, and saliva, people caring for victims are particularly at risk, especially family members. Fortunately, it is not believed that Ebola can be spread from human to human by airborne transmission, which helps with containment. Many health-care workers, in spite of what was thought to be optimal protection, still caught the virus and died.

- The number of viral particles in one drop of blood is more than a million times greater than HIV, which increases its contagion capacity. This led to a huge increase in the production of protective garments, boots, masks, and gloves, known as personal protective equipment.

- Hospitals in the United States increased their supplies of protective gear and provided training to first-line staff on how to put it on and take it off safely. Financial support from other countries allowed the purchase of similar equipment for affected countries.

MERS and SARS

- Middle East respiratory syndrome (MERS) first surfaced in the Middle East in 2012 in Jordan, and most cases have occurred in the Arabian Peninsula. With new viruses like MERS emerging, and our experience with Ebola in the United States, stringent protocols have been put in place by the Centers for Disease Control and Prevention (CDC) to rapidly diagnose these patients and contain the illnesses. In addition, the CDC continues to upgrade the preparedness for airline and airport staff, who are crucial to the containment efforts.

- About a decade has passed since the original severe acute respiratory syndrome (SARS) outbreak of 2003. Although there were only eight confirmed cases of SARS in the United States, there were more than 8,000 global cases with almost a 50 percent death rate.

- Both the SARS and MERS viruses are part of the *Coronavirus* family. Coronaviruses are known for the crown-like spikes on their surfaces. The virus causes disease in the lungs and a bloody pneumonia. Importantly, coronaviruses can remain suspended in the air and travel more than eight feet. They can be transmitted from person to person.

- The World Health Organization (WHO) is concerned about MERS. We don't know what the reservoir is or how it's transmitted. An unlikely animal reservoir was discovered in Saudi Arabia: a camel. However, it is unclear if the camel is actually the direct source of the virus or just a vector of transmission to humans. The other postulated reservoir is bats.

- The WHO is particularly worried about opportunities for spread of the virus among large communities and large gatherings. Fortunately, they are better prepared to deal with MERS because of their experience with its cousin, SARS.

- Because of the intense coordination and collaboration efforts between countries during the SARS outbreak, they were able to contain the virus. Containment of the disease was possible because the incubation period of both these viruses is about 10 to 14 days, and old-fashioned quarantine was successful.

- There is no vaccine or any specific treatment for MERS or SARS. The WHO also implemented reporting requirements and early identification measures for MERS. For now, monitoring will continue to ensure that everything is in place to prevent an epidemic, and scientists will continue to study the virus and its transmission.

West Nile Virus

- West Nile virus was first detected in the United States in 1999, although it was found in Israel in the 1950s and spread throughout Europe, North Africa, and Asia over the next decades.

- After being bitten by an infected mosquito, surprisingly more than half of all infected people are completely asymptomatic. Those who are symptomatic usually have a high fever and muscle aches for 48 hours—similar to, but not as severe as, dengue—with resolution of the illness over the next few days. However, those over the age of 50 are more prone to neurological symptoms that may include meningitis or even encephalitis and could result in death. Fortunately, this occurrence is rare.

- One the most identifiable birds in the United States, the American robin, was found to be one of the most prevalent carriers of West Nile virus. Mosquitoes serve as the vector of the disease: They bite the robin, which harbors the virus without symptoms and then passes it on to humans without mosquito protection.

- One thing you can do for your community is report dead birds to your state health department. This helps the surveillance efforts to monitor where possible disease outbreaks might occur.

Chikungunya

- Chikungunya is a viral disease transmitted to humans by the bites of infected mosquitoes found across the globe. First described during an outbreak in southern Tanzania in 1952, the virus then spread to Africa, Asia, and the Indian subcontinent. Originally believed to be a tropical disease, experts were surprised when an outbreak occurred in northeastern Italy in 2007.

- Now it has spread further—to 14 Caribbean island countries since it was first detected on the island of Saint Martin in December of 2013. In May of 2014, the Caribbean Public Health Authority declared it an epidemic, with more than 5,000 probable cases across the region. Its symptoms are very similar to dengue viral infection, although it may not be as severe and deaths are exceedingly unusual.

- Because the Caribbean islands are close to the United States, the virus made its premiere appearance in the United States in 2014. The CDC has been working with its partners at airports with flights to the Caribbean to educate outgoing travelers about how to stay safe from chikungunya and to alert returning travelers about what symptoms to be on the lookout for.

Reemerging Diseases

- New diseases aren't popping up as fast as the reappearance of old diseases that were nearly eradicated. Reemerging diseases are due to many human factors, such as technology, social behavior, and international travel and trade.

- For example, measles was declared eradicated in the United States in 2000, yet measles and mumps are on the rise. Some people contracted these diseases because they were either unvaccinated or not up to date with their immunizations and encountered someone—perhaps while traveling—who had measles. Because measles is one of the most contagious diseases due to its airborne capacity, this is a growing concern.

- While vaccination deficiencies can also lead to mumps, the mumps virus has mutated enough that the original vaccine does not have 100 percent protection. It is estimated that the mumps vaccine is only 80 to 90 percent effective. Several college campuses are seeing outbreaks of mumps, and now most colleges require proof of vaccination for incoming students.

- Pertussis, or whooping cough, was never eliminated in the United States, unlike measles and polio, so it surfaces from time to time. However, the incidence is increasing. From an immunological standpoint, this might be because, in the 1990s, the United States switched from the DTP to the DTaP, which contains a modified, safer version of the pertussis vaccine, eliminating the risk of seizures. It is postulated that this new vaccine does not last as long as the old one, so our protection wanes more quickly over the years.

- A relatively current national recommendation is for all adults over the age of 50, and especially those over 60 who are in contact with infants, to get a pertussis booster vaccine as part of the DTaP vaccine. Adults experiencing immune senescence will reacquire immunity and prevent transmission to vulnerable children under one year of age, who may die from pertussis.

- All three of these diseases—measles, mumps, and pertussis—are carefully monitored by the CDC, so they are aware of any changes that might be concerning to the U.S. population. In addition, scientists are continually working to improve vaccines. Recommended child, young adult, and adult boosters are listed on a schedule on the CDC site.

Chronic Diseases

- Scientists think it is possible that chronic diseases might actually stem from an infectious cause. It's possible that we might be able to cure chronic diseases, such as heart disease, with an antibiotic. Further studies into whether other diseases might also stem from infectious roots have turned our thinking upside down. This has major implications for the diagnosis and treatment of disease in the future.

- Presently, there are several chronic medical conditions that might be caused by a known infectious agent and other illnesses from unknown infectious organisms yet to be discovered. Some conditions under investigation include coronary artery disease, inflammatory bowel disease, arthritis conditions, diabetes, and even some neurological disorders.

- Sometimes the microorganism can be the direct cause of the disease, while other times the germ could incite an autoimmune body reaction. Interactions between humans and microorganisms are wondrous and complex. Extraordinary changes will continue to occur over time in our understanding of infectious diseases.

Suggested Reading

Garrett, *The Coming Plague*.

Karlen, *Man and Microbes*.

Preston, *The Hot Zone*.

Questions to Consider

1. Why do there continue to be new infectious diseases, and why are some old ones making a comeback? Do you expect this trend to continue?

2. The Ebola virus outbreak in Africa was very scary to hear about. Is an Ebola or similar outbreak in the United States likely? What might prevent it?

Outbreak! Contagion! The Next Pandemic!

Lecture 24

How worried should we be about the next pandemic being one deadly enough to cause hundreds of thousands of deaths worldwide, spreading through countries, leaping across oceans, and overwhelming entire continents? This lecture will look into the future to try to discern what the next pandemic will be, based on the variables that create a pandemic and disease control issues. The focus is not on just a pandemic confined to a few countries but a cataclysmic pandemic—one that would reach all continents quickly, be difficult to treat, be extremely deadly, and perhaps threaten the very survival of the human race.

Historical Lessons from Past Pandemics

- The historical lessons from pandemics of the past can help us determine what the next one might be. There have been seven cholera pandemics, including the latest one, which has been ongoing for more than 50 years. Cholera is caused by the *Vibrio cholera* bacteria, which releases potent toxins resulting in severe diarrhea. The first cholera pandemic was documented in 1816 in Bengal, India, and the latest one started in 1962 in Indonesia.

- There have been several pandemics attributed to plague, which is a vector-borne disease that is spread by the bite of fleas that feed on rodents infected with *Yersinia pestis*, also a bacteria. Sporadic cases still occur in the United States, and nearly 100 cases erupted in Madagascar in 2014.

- There have been four influenza pandemics in the last century: the 1918 Spanish flu, the 1957 Asian flu, the 1968 Hong Kong flu, and the swine flu variant in Mexico in 2009—all of which were the result of reassorted viruses.

- Cholera, plague, and influenza have been wreaking havoc for many years. What factors have changed since the 19th and 20th centuries that might influence our pandemic possibilities? Are these older pandemic germs now under control? We now have better control of diseases, at least in some areas. For example, we have better diagnostics and treatments, new vaccines, better protective equipment (such as gloves and masks), improved funding from global sources, and global surveillance systems that coordinate responses.

The Next Pandemic

- A pandemic could occur at any time. It most likely would start in Southeast or East Asia. Transmission will likely be aerosol and airborne. Tick- and vector- borne diseases are unlikely. Certain bacteria are possible, but less likely.

- If it's viral, it will likely be an RNA virus with a single-stranded genome, because RNA viruses replicate even faster than DNA ones. Many of the new emerging and reemerging diseases are RNA viruses.

- Ebola can be spread by close contact or blood, but, like anthrax, it is likely too efficient at causing deaths, meaning that people aren't traveling long distances when they are that ill—in fact, they're dying so the spread is more contained. In developed countries, with a 3- to 21-day incubation period, quarantine measures may be effective.

- The coronaviruses SARS and MERS are good candidates, because they are easily transmitted, have a modest mortality rate, and have no known effective antiviral medications. However, the incubation period is 4 to 7 days for coronaviruses, so patients can be isolated and transmission can be disrupted. This is how the original SARS was contained. So, maybe we'll reduce the chances of SARS and MERS for now because we may be able to contain them.

- Measles and mumps are on the list, but they are unlikely unless there is a significant mutation in childhood viruses that would render current vaccines ineffective.

- Smallpox could be a problem due to its ease of transmission, its high mortality rate, and because there is virtually no natural human immunity to previous virus exposures. But we'll consider it less likely because there are no natural reservoirs in the world, and we already have a vaccine and are working on improving laboratory safety.

- Developed countries have a better chance of stemming HIV infections, with cutting-edge diagnostics and drugs. This will most probably remain a deadly killer in developing countries.

- It is likely that influenza will be the cause of the next cataclysmic pandemic—possibly H5N1 or other varieties of avian influenza, such as H7N9. Influenza has already been implicated in four pandemics in the last 100 years. It has a short 48- to 72-hour incubation period, so those infected have already transmitted the virus before they know that they are sick. It's also tough to implement quarantine with this short time window.

- Influenza makes people ill, but it usually doesn't kill them, so people are carrying the virus at various stages of their illness and could infect many others. Influenza can mutate rapidly and undergo antigenic drift or shift.

- Fortunately, so far, avian influenza H5N1 strain does not transmit easily between humans because certain throat cell receptors are missing. However, in the 600 cases that occurred in 15 different countries, 60 percent died, so this could be a force to be reckoned with. Most of these cases were the result of direct contact with infected poultry.

- Asia, with its large poultry markets, continues to be closely watched for outbreaks of avian influenza H5N1—particularly Laos, which has had an outbreak of this virus every year since 2006. China has seen the emergence of the deadly H7N9 avian virus that could be especially deadly because it is made up of four different avian flu viruses from a wild duck, a wild bird, and two species of chickens.

- The current world population has not had much exposure to the avian flu variants, so there is little immunity. All that these viruses would need to become a pandemic is an enhanced capacity to transmit from human to human, or resistance capacity to all current antiviral medications, or both.

- We are fortunate that avian influenza is still sensitive to neuraminidase drugs, but would there be enough to go around? Because influenza can mutate so rapidly, we would also need a new vaccine to be produced quickly and made readily available worldwide.

- With the 1918 flu pandemic, many of the deaths resulted from a secondary infection from bacterial pneumonia. We now have antibiotics, but the idea of co-pathogens playing an additional role in the pandemic must be considered.

- A strain of Avian influenza—or an unknown emerging zoonotic virus—are the most likely future culprits of a pandemic, but smallpox could surprise us, and bacteria resistant to all antibiotics might not be far behind.

In Pandemic Mode

- Assuming that we are in pandemic mode, there are three more questions that directly affect you.
    - How would people find out about the pandemic?

    - How long would it take to develop an antidote or vaccine?

    - What can you do to prepare yourself and your family?

- New technologies would be helpful in an outbreak situation. The following are all good sources, depending your daily life habits.
    - mHealth, an alert by the latest, most innovative wireless mobile health technology

    - A Google Flu Trends report on the Internet

- The Outbreaks Near Me app
- A Facebook posting or a Twitter tweet
- The regular news media

- To help out, there are several worldwide disease alert systems already in place, and most will accept information incoming from any source—individual or otherwise. Canada's Global Public Health Intelligence Network uses automated, aggregated news feeds based on search queries and was the first to identify the SARS outbreak in 2003, even before the World Health Organization's (WHO) report, which came out months later. Because of early detection, they were able to contain the outbreak.

- A collaborative network of many world health organizations known as the Global Early Warning System exists to improve early warning and risk assessment on zoonoses and emerging infectious diseases. Google and Yahoo are using keyword search queries to determine whether this type of collective intelligence gathering could predict outbreaks. One thing we can predict is that technology will continue to evolve just as fast as diseases.

- How long would it take to find an antidote/vaccine if it is a new disease? It used to take a decade or more to get vaccines through the rigorous requirements of the FDA. With a global health crisis, it has been reduced to four to six months, depending on the pathogen. But this means that those populations affected early in the pandemic will not have an available vaccine and will have to rely on current medications and supportive care.

- The 2014 Ebola outbreak in West Africa was a game-changing instance where rules got broken. Extraordinary measures were taken by the NIH during this outbreak to accelerate the timeline for FDA approval of a clinical trial for a vaccine. This became a matter of moral duty—with drugs not tested and proven through lengthy clinical trials for effectiveness and safety.

- Another rule-breaking decision was made by WHO's panel of ethicists, who were in unanimous agreement to offer untested treatments. One example of this is ZMapp, a drug that had been in development for more than 10 years but was not safety tested. It was given to two Americans who contracted Ebola in Africa and were flown to the United States for treatment. The Americans recovered, but other patients who were given the same drug died. Unfortunately, the drug was only available in a tiny quantity, though, and because it was produced in genetically engineered tobacco plants, it would take months to make more of it.

Protecting Yourself and Your Family

- Obviously, staying away from sick people is just good common sense. Putting together an emergency kit and stocking up on food and water and supplies would be helpful, and so would getting an approved N95 mask that can filter small particles, bacteria, and viruses.

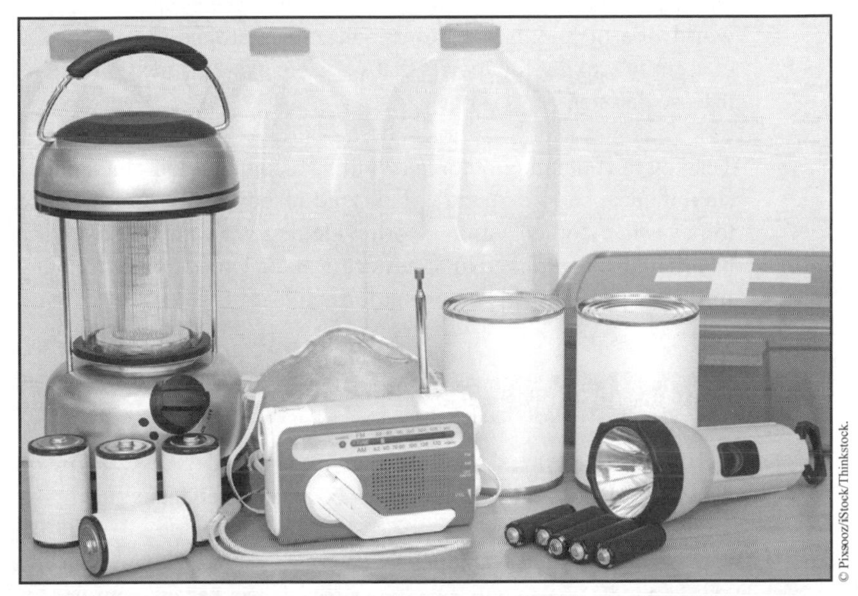

In case of an emergency, you should have a supply of items you might need, such as batteries, flashlights, lanterns, a first aid kit, a radio, bottled water, and cans of food.

- Scientists predict that in the event of a cataclysmic pandemic, airline travel would shut down, international trade would be curtailed, and Internet access might be limited or fail. Can you imagine the economic impact this would have? Every business should have a preparedness plan in place that would enable people to telecommute and still keep business going. The flu.gov site has a great Business Preparedness Checklist to help you get organized.

- The future of infectious diseases is one of rapid changes. Infectious diseases can evolve rapidly, but our knowledge of disease causes and treatments is also evolving. Whirlwind developments in technological advances improve both our capability for diagnosis and treatment, as well as our ability to detect outbreaks before they get out of control.

- In an ever-changing world where humans are overrunning animal habitats—where diseases are jumping onto planes and spreading worldwide in a matter of hours—scientists around the world are constantly looking for signals that will help avert the next infectious disease disaster.

- The key to containing outbreaks will be a combination of enhanced surveillance, early detection, and rapid response. We are fortunate to have many organizations worldwide that are watching over our health in this regard and to have access in the United States to many forms of technology to keep us informed.

Questions to Consider

1. Do you really think it is possible that there could be a worldwide cataclysmic infectious disease event that could threaten mankind?

2. What are the most likely possibilities for such a pandemic, and how can you and your family be prepared in case such an event ever began to unfold?

Bibliography

Abbas, Abul, Andrew Lichtman, and Shiv Pillai. *Basic Immunology: Functions and Disorders of the Immune System*. Philadelphia: Elsevier-Saunders, 2012. This concise, focused text provides you with an introduction to the workings of the human immune system.

Atlas, Ronald, and Stanley Maloy. *One Health: People, Animals, and the Environment*. Washington, DC: ASM Press, 2014. This book presents core concepts of links between human and animal health. It also cites remaining challenges of One Health to preventing the threat of emerging infectious disease. The book will provide a series of stories about how disruption of the environment and transmission from animal hosts is responsible for emerging human and animal diseases.

Barry, John M. *The Great Influenza: The Epic Story of the Deadliest Plague in History*. New York: Viking, 2004. This book focuses not only on the science and epidemiology behind one of the worst pandemics of all time, but also on the effects of disease outbreaks during wartime.

Blaser, Martin J. *Missing Microbes*. New York: Henry Holt and Company, 2014. Both a primer on microbiology as well as an in-depth presentation of how the overuse of antibiotics in patients, and in our food supplies, has negatively affected public health. Discussion on the human gastrointestinal microbiome and links to the obesity epidemic.

Booss, John, and Marilyn J. August. *To Catch a Virus*. Washington, DC: ASM Press, 2013. Presents the historical discovery of viruses, the pioneers of viral research, and the evolution of the field up to current technologies, including molecular and genetic techniques.

Bud, Robert. *Penicillin: Triumph and Tragedy*. New York: Oxford University Press, 2007. A well-written and authoritative history of the discovery, application, and importance of penicillin and the evolution of resistant microbes. Includes the impact that penicillin has had on modern-day life.

Byerly, C. R. *Fever of War: The Influenza Epidemic in the U.S. Army During World War I*. New York: New York University Press, 2005. Having collected diaries and mementos of soldiers, Byerly presents the substantial impact that the flu pandemic of 1918 had on the U.S. Army and how the crowded conditions of war provides the perfect environment for disease.

Cave, Stephanie. *What Your Doctor May Not Tell You about Children's Vaccinations*. New York: Grand Central Life and Style, 2010. A well-written guide for parents about vaccinations. Pros and cons of vaccines are discussed to help parents make a knowledgeable choice about vaccinating their children.

Cole, Leonard A. *Clouds of Secrecy: The Army's Germ Warfare Tests over Populated Areas*. Totowa, NJ: Rowman & Littlefield, 1999. An insightful description of the secret tests that were done by the U.S. Army in the 1970s to study the effects of biological weapons.

Crawford, Dorothy H. *Deadly Companions: How Microbes Shaped Our History*. New York: Oxford University Press, 2007. A study of the evolution of microbes and how they continue to challenge scientists with their ability to cause disease. Crawford also analyzes how microbes have adapted to changes in society, from hunter-gatherers to modern-day cities and global travelers.

———. *The Invisible Enemy: A Natural History of Viruses*. New York: Oxord University Press, 2000. An introduction to the world of viruses, including their history and evolution, as well as how we have dealt with the continuing challenges of mutations.

Crosby, Alfred W. *America's Forgotten Pandemic: The Influenza of 1918*. 2nd ed. New York: Cambridge University Press, 2003. Previously published as *Epidemic and Peace, 1918* (1976), this book revives interest in the pandemic of 1918 and its affects on humans then, as well as its relevance in medicine today.

———. *The Columbian Exchange: Biological and Cultural Consequences of 1492*. 30th anniversary ed. Westport, CT: Praeger, 2003. A fascinating analysis of the impact of Columbus's voyage in terms of the biological exchanges between the old and new worlds. This included not only the exchange of plants and animals but also pathogens.

De Kruif, Paul. *Microbe Hunters*. New York: Harcourt, Brace and Company, 1926. A solid account of the first bacteriologists and other scientists who were involved in the discovery of bacteria and who worked on vaccines to control them.

Diamond, Jared M. *Guns, Germs, and Steel: The Fates of Human Societies*. New York: W. W. Norton & Company, 2005. Written through the eyes of a geography professor, this book is a great presentation on how the modern world evolved since the ice age—in terms of demography, ecology, and geography. He theorizes that the pace of development of civilizations were more likely due to biological differences rather than races and defines the impact germs had.

Garrett, Laurie. *The Coming Plague: Newly Emerging Diseases in a World Out of Balance*. New York: Farrar, Straus and Giroux, 1994. The story of how changing social and environmental conditions has resulted in emerging, reemerging, and often deadly infectious diseases. Garrett is the only writer to have been awarded the Peabody, Polk, and Pulitzer.

Gaynes, Robert P. *Germ Theory: Medical Pioneers in Infectious Diseases*. Washington, DC: ASM Press, 2011. The stories of medical pioneers who changed the world of infectious diseases and contributed to the understanding of germ theory, starting with Hippocrates.

Gladwin, Mark, and Bill Trattler. *Clinical Microbiology Made Ridiculously Simple*. 6th ed. Miami, FL: Medmaster, 2014. A great resource to better understand the principles of microbiology in a humorous and easy-to-learn fashion. This edition includes updates on *C. difficile*, HIV treatments, pandemic flu concerns, and drug-resistant TB.

Grossman, Leigh. *Infection Control in the Child Care Center and Preschool*. New York: Demos Publishing, 2012. The handbook covers both common and unusual infections and illnesses prevalent in this population and offers practical guidance on issues of contagion, treatment, and transmission. This handbook is the most recognized for best practices for treating and preventing the spread of infection in children in daycare and preschool.

Hager, Thomas. *The Demon under the Microscope: From Battlefield Hospitals to Nazi Labs, One Doctor's Heroic Search for the World's First Miracle Drug*. New York: Harmony Books, 2006. A riveting story about the development of the first antibiotic: sulfa. This sparked a new era in the development of other drugs, as well as the first ability to treat numerous deadly bacterial infections.

Harper, David R., and Andrea S. Meyer. *Of Mice, Men and Microbes: Hantavirus*. San Diego: Academic Press, 1999. This book describes the first deadly infections of the hantavirus in 1993 in the southwestern United States. It also explains why there is no treatment, cure, or vaccine for this deadly virus.

Harrison, Mark. *Contagion: How Commerce Has Spread Disease*. New Haven: Yale University Press, 2012. The author demonstrates in this book how over time, commerce has spread, and continues to spread, diseases worldwide. It starts in the 14th century with plagues in Eurasia, and then discusses the development over time of the public health system and insinuates that we should not get comfortable with our ability to conquer all germs.

Henderson, Donald A. *Smallpox: The Death of a Disease—The Inside Story of Eradicating a Worldwide Killer*. Amherst, NY: Prometheus Books, 2009. A fascinating personal story of Dr. Henderson's efforts with the World Heath Organization to eradicate smallpox and the barriers and obstacles they faced in the process. He includes the complex issues of whether to destroy remaining stores of smallpox or not.

Karlen, Arno. *Man and Microbes: Disease and Plagues in History and Modern Times*. New York: Simon & Schuster, 1996. Arno attempts to answer the questions of where new diseases come from and why old diseases are reemerging. He looks at the coevolution of humans and microbes and how socioecological changes have affected the rise of diseases. He puts the blame squarely on our environmental challenges and our behavior.

Kauffman, Carol, Peter Pappas, Jack Sobel, and William Dismukes. *Essentials of Clinical Mycology*. 2nd ed. New York: Springer, 2011. A comprehensive textbook covering the classification of all fungal diseases. Includes the epidemiology of endemic mycosis, such as blastomycosis and histoplasmosis. Also discusses antifungal therapy.

Hall, Brian, and John Hall. *Skin Infections: Diagnosis and Treatment*. New York: Cambridge University Press, 2009. This book attempts to integrate the medical specialties of infectious diseases and dermatology. The book is organized into types of infections, locations of infection by skin layer, and specific populations of patients at risk.

Lax, Eric. *The Mold in Dr. Florey's Coat: The Story of the Penicillin Miracle*. New York: Henry Holt and Company, 2004. This is the story of how penicillin inadvertently arrived in a London laboratory in 1928, becoming one of the most important drugs in history. This is also the story of how it was not just one man's efforts to succeed at this discovery and gives credit to three others who were significantly involved in the effort and describes the difficulty of working in war conditions.

Leavitt, Judith Walzer. *Typhoid Mary: Captive to the Public's Health*. Boston: Beacon Press, 1996. The story of an Irish immigrant cook in the early 1900s who infected 22 people with typhoid fever through her food.

Levy, Stuart B. *The Antibiotic Paradox: How Miracle Drugs Are Destroying the Miracle*. New York: Plenum, 1992. Levy describes the overuse of antibiotics and the peril it is causing in treating current diseases.

Mangold, Tom, and Jeff Goldberg. *Plague Wars: A True Story of Biological Warfare*. New York: St. Martin's Press, 2000. Mangold gives us a terrifying look at current biowarfare that is going on across the world in secret.

Margulis, Lynn, and Dorion Sagan. *Microcosmos: Four Billion Years of Microbial Evolution*. Berkeley: University of California Press, 1997. A complex description of how the contributions of microorganisms affect the evolution of life on our planet. The authors also discuss the significant role of symbiosis in cell evolution, rather than mutation of bacteria as the determinant of change on Earth.

Marrie, Thomas. *Community-Acquired Pneumonia*. New York: Kluwer Academic and Plenum Publishers, 2014. This book is designed to review the causes of community-acquired pneumonia and to identify critical questions in the 21st century that will help us better understand this condition.

McNeill, William Hardy. *Plagues and Peoples*. Garden City, NY: Anchor Press, 1976. A survey of the impact of infectious diseases on history in terms of human evolution and our ability to thrive in the face of exposure to new diseases.

Morris, J. Glenn, and Potter Morris. *Foodborne Infections and Intoxications*. New York: Academic Press and Elselvier, 2013. This book covers the impact of food-borne diseases and intoxications. The accelerated globalization of the food supply is also discussed.

Nuland, Sherwin B. *The Doctors' Plague: Germs, Childbed Fever, and the Strange Story of Ignaz Semmelweis*. Great Discoveries. Reprint ed. New York: W. W. Norton & Company, 2004. The story of how Semmelweis saved many pregnant women from death by implementing hand-washing procedures in 1847. Unfortunately, his colleagues refused to believe in his theories, and he endured their criticisms until his death.

O'Shea, Tim. *Vaccination Is Not Immunization*. San Antonio: Immunition Ltd, 2013. This book examines each vaccine separately, including the history of the vaccination, incidence of the disease, and side effects. It gives parents the tools required to make decisions regarding which vaccinations they feel comfortable with, when to vaccinate, when not to vaccinate, and why. This vaccine book is written in an easy-to-understand language. This is not an anti-vaccine book. This book is in favor of any vaccines that have been found to be effective with little chance of harm to the recipient.

Oshinsky, David M. *Polio: An American Story—The Crusade That Mobilized the Nation against the 20th Century's Most Feared Disease*. Oxford: Oxford University Press, 2005. A good historical book that gives insight into what it took to discover a vaccine to keep thousands of people from dying of polio in the United States. It also gives insight into the competition between Jonas Salk and Albert Sabin as they each tried to make the discovery first.

Preston, Richard. *The Hot Zone*. New York: Random House, 1994. The terrifying story of the Ebola outbreak in a lab in Reston, Virginia.

Quammen, David. *Spillover: Animal Infections and the Next Human Pandemic*. New York: W. W. Norton & Company, 2012. A description of the leap of animal- and insect-borne diseases to humans, including how to trace diseases to animals, as well as methods of transmission and mutations. Quammen details how changes in the environment affect disease transmission and spread and relates how intricately we are linked to the entire web of the Earth's ecosystems.

Rotbart, Harley. *Germ Proof Your Kids: The Complete Guide to Protecting (without Overprotecting) Your Family from Infections*. Washington, DC: ASM Press, 2007. A practical reference written by an infectious disease specialist that portrays both the myths associated with germs and the science behind the explanation. Written for adults but also at an instructional level that will enable you to teach family and children.

Ryan, Frank. *The Forgotten Plague*. Boston: Little, Brown & Company, 1992. Dr. Ryan reminds us not to forget tuberculosis—a disease of the past, but one that is still virulent today. It has increased its relevance by becoming resistant, in forms, to antibiotics. He traces the history of TB, the search for a cure, and the issues that confront us today.

Sachs, Jessica Snyder. *Good Germs, Bad Germs: Health and Survival in a Bacterial World*. New York: Hill and Wang, 2007. Antibiotics have unintentionally disrupted the balance between humans and the microorganisms that inhabit our bodies and our environment. As a result, antibiotic resistance issues are top priorities for the Centers for Disease

Control and Prevention and the World Heath Organization. This book tells the story of what went wrong in our war on germs.

Shah, Sonia. *The Fever: How Malaria Has Ruled Humankind for 500,000 Years*. New York: Farrar, Straus and Giroux, 2010. The complete story of malaria, from the ancient to the modern world. This includes stories of how malaria changed history.

Sherman, Irwin W. *Twelve Diseases That Changed Our World*. Washington, DC: ASM Press, 2007. An excellent summary of the author's top 12 list of infectious diseases that had the most impact on the modern era of human history.

Shilts, Randy. *And the Band Played On: Politics, People, and the AIDS Epidemic*. Rev. ed. New York: St. Martin's Griffin, 2007. The story of a gay airline steward who allegedly was responsible for a large portion of the early spread of HIV. The book then discusses the politics of HIV in the 1980s and the lack of U.S. government effort in facilitating medical developments due to HIV's ties with the gay community.

Spreen, Kathleen. *Compendium of Tick-Borne Disease: A Thousand Pearls*. Pocopson, PA: Pocopson Publishing LLC, 2013. A comprehensive overview of tick-borne diseases, including Lyme disease, Ehrlichia, and anaplasma. The text was designed to educate patients about the risks posed by tick-borne illnesses. The author dispels harmful myths and provides a solid scientific foundation for the practical guidance to tick-borne diseases.

Skloot, Rebecca. *The Immortal Life of Henrietta Lacks*. New York: Broadway Books, 2011. The story of how a woman's unfortunate cancer diagnosis became one of the biggest gifts to science, sparking innovations in cancer treatments, gene mapping, vaccines, and more.

Sompayrac, Lauren. *How the Immune System Works*. Hoboken, NJ: Wiley Blackwell, 2012. The book contains 15 easy-to-follow lectures that provide an introduction to immunology, followed by a practical discussion on how each of the components interacts with one another. The author reveals in simple language the essence of this complex subject.

Vincent, Jean-Louis, Jean Carlet, and Steven Opal. *The Sepsis Text*. Norwell, MA: Kluwer Academic Publishers, 2014. This comprehensive textbook on sepsis gives a perspective on the multitude of laboratory research, including the physiological processes and antisepsis therapies.

Waksman, Selman A. *The Conquest of Tuberculosis*. London: University of California Press, 1964. This book tells the story of the discovery of the first TB drug: streptomycin.

Weston, Debbie. *Fundamentals of Infection Prevention and Control: Theory and Practice*. Hoboken: Wiley and Sons, 2013. This book gives readers the essentials of the principles of infection control. It provides a comprehensive guide to the prevention, management, and control of health-care–associated infections. It discusses the basic elements of microbiology, immunology, and epidemiology that underlie hospital-related infections.

Zimmer, Carl. *A Planet of Viruses*. Chicago: University of Chicago Press, 2012. A short review of the history and ubiquity of viruses throughout the world.

Zinsser, Hans. *Rats, Lice and History*. Boston: Atlantic Monthly Press, 1935. Originally written in 1935 by Zinsser, the goal of the book was to bring science, philosophy, and literature together to establish the importance of disease—and especially epidemic infectious disease—as a major force in human affairs. This book is devoted to a discussion of the biology of typhus and history of typhus fever in human affairs.

Organizations

Centers for Disease Control and Prevention (CDC)
CDC.gov

This site has a wealth of information and literature related to infectious diseases that includes tabs for Diseases and Conditions, Healthy Living, and Travelers' Health. It also includes links to its scientific publication, the *Morbidity and Mortality Weekly Report*, and other topics, such as global health and publications, and even a Solve the Outbreak app!

Also, check the following page for information on the latest health news and for how to make an emergency kit.

http://emergency.cdc.gov/preparedness/kit/disasters/

Other CDC Web References

1918 influenza pandemic (Lecture 21)

wwwnc.cdc.gov/eid/article/12/1/pdfs/05-0979.pdf

Antimicrobial stewardship and improved antibiotic use (Lecture 17)

http://www.cdc.gov/getsmart/healthcare/implementation/core-elements.html

http://www.cdc.gov/mmwr/preview/mmwrhtml/mm6309a4.htm?s_cid=mm6309a4_w

Antibiotic resistance threats in the United States (Lecture 6)

http://www.cdc.gov/drugresistance/threat-report-2013/pdf/ar-threats-2013-508.pdf

Avian influenza (Lecture 21, 24)

http://www.cdc.gov/flu/avianflu/h5n1-people.htm

http://www.cdc.gov/flu/avianflu/h7n9-virus.htm

Botulism toxin (Lecture 22)

www.bt.cdc.gov/agent/botulism/botulismconsensus.pdf

Emergency preparedness and response (Lecture 22)

http://www.bt.cdc.gov/bioterrorism/

Emerging Infectious Diseases

http://wwwnc.cdc.gov/eid/

This peer-reviewed, open-access journal is published monthly by the CDC. It provides current information on new and emerging infectious diseases and their global impact.

1918 influenza revisited (Lecture 21)

http://wwwnc.cdc.gov/eid/article/12/1/05-1442_article

Reflections on the 1976 swine flu vaccination (Lecture 21)

http://wwwnc.cdc.gov/eid/article/12/1/05-1007-t1

Epidemics after natural disasters (Lecture 20)

http://wwwnc.cdc.gov/eid/article/13/1/06-0779_article.htm#r26

Fungal meningitis (Lecture 4)

http://www.cdc.gov/hai/outbreaks/meningitis.html

Get Smart about Antibiotics (Lecture 6)

http://www.cdc.gov/getsmart/

Hepatitis (Lecture 8)

http://www.cdc.gov/hepatitis/index.htm

HIV

http://www.cdc.gov/hiv/default.html (Lecture 18)

Immunizations and recommended vaccination schedules (Lecture 9)

http://www.cdc.gov/vaccines/acip/

Middle East respiratory syndrome (MERS) (Lecture 23)

http://www.cdc.gov/coronavirus/mers/US.html

National Center for Emerging and Zoonotic Diseases (Lecture 11, 12, 23)

http://www.cdc.gov/ncezid/index.html

A unit of the CDC, this center focuses on prevention of infectious diseases, incorporating the One Health Initiative strategy to improve human and animal health, as well as improve our environment. This site has a Current Outbreak List, the *Emerging Infectious Diseases* journal, a section on innovative technologies, and many articles applicable to daily life. This site also includes links to its other divisions, such as Preparedness and Emerging Infections and Foodborne, Waterborne, and Environmental Diseases.

Norovirus food-borne outbreaks (Lecture 1, 8)

http://www.cdc.gov/mmwr/preview/mmwrhtml/mm6322a3.htm?s_cid=mm6322a3_w

Reality of outbreak investigation and pandemics (Lecture 24)

http://blogs.cdc.gov/publichealthmatters/2013/07/dengue-in-angola/

Sexually transmitted diseases (Lecture 16)

http://www.cdc.gov/std/

Sporotrichosis outbreak (Lecture 4)

http://www.cdc.gov/mmwr/preview/mmwrhtml/00001173.htm

Surveillance for travel-related diseases (Geosentinel Surveillance System) (Lecture 20)

http://www.cdc.gov/mmwr/preview/mmwrhtml/ss6203a1.htm

Travel precautions, vaccinations, and health alerts (Lecture 20)

http://wwwnc.cdc.gov/travel

http://wwwnc.cdc.gov/travel/yellowbook/2014/appendices/appendix-d-the-healthmap-system

Food and Drug Administration (FDA)

Animal antibiotic use summary report (Lecture 6)

http://www.fda.gov/downloads/forindustry/userfees/animaldruguserfeeactADUFA/UCM338170.pdf

Vaccine for H5N1 influenza (Lecture 21, 24)

http://www.fda.gov/newsevents/newsroom/pressannouncements/ucm376444.htm

Gates Foundation and Global Health

http://www.gatesfoundation.org/What-We-Do

While the foundation focuses on different issues, such as poverty, health, and education, its Global Health arm funds many innovative research projects to improve health worldwide. This site demonstrates the depth of the international partnerships they have and the wide range of research projects they fund.

Google (Lecture 24)
Google.org

This is the philanthropic arm of the Internet search company that funds various types of projects worldwide, including the use of its search engine and Google Earth to improve global health.

http://singularityhub.com/2014/09/14/predicting-and-preventing-the-spread-of-infectious-disease-with-google-earth/

http://wwwnc.cdc.gov/eid/article/15/8/09-0299_article

http://www.microbemagazine.org/index.php?option=com_content&view=article&id=84:google-underwrites-several-infectious-disease-surveillance-efforts&catid=46&Itemid=187

HealthMap (Lecture 20)
http://healthmap.org/site/about

This is the site of the developers of the Outbreaks Near Me app, which uses informal sources and partners to identify disease outbreaks and was developed in 2006 by a team of epidemiologists, researchers, and software developers at Boston Children's Hospital. This site also offers a wide range of scholarly articles.

The Kaiser Family Foundation (Lecture 18, 19)
http://kff.org/global-health-policy/

This foundation is a resource for a variety of global health issues, both in the United States and abroad, including malaria, TB, and HIV/AIDS. This site also provides summary information on health-care policies, funding, and current health issues.

National Center for Biotechnology
www.ncbi.nlm.nih.gov/

Through this site, you can access many books and articles with their Bookshelf feature—some of which are interlinked with PubMed.

Armed conflict and infectious diseases (Lecture 20)

http://www.ncbi.nlm.nih.gov/books/NBK45724/

Early detection of outbreaks using the Internet (Lecture 24)

http://www.ncbi.nlm.nih.gov/pmc/articles/PMC2665960/

Emerging and reemerging diseases (Lecture 23)

http://www.ncbi.nlm.nih.gov/books/NBK20370/

Exercise and the immune system (Lecture 10)

http://www.nlm.nih.gov/medlineplus/ency/article/007165.htm

Globalization of the food supply (Lecture 13)

http://www.ncbi.nlm.nih.gov/books/NBK45724/

Global travel and trade (Lecture 20, 23)

http://www.ncbi.nlm.nih.gov/books/NBK45724/

Origins of HIV (Lecture 18)

http://www.ncbi.nlm.nih.gov/pmc/articles/PMC3234451/

Travel, conflict, trade, and disease (Lecture 20)

http://www.ncbi.nlm.nih.gov/books/NBK45724/

National Institute of Allergy and Infectious Diseases (NIAID)
http://www.niaid.nih.gov

This branch of the National Institutes of Health funds research to prevent and treat infectious (and other) diseases. This has resulted in new treatments, vaccines, and technologies that have improved health care worldwide.

The immune system (Lecture 10)

http://www.niaid.nih.gov/topics/immunesystem/Pages/default.aspx

Vaccine development: HIV (Lecture 18)

http://www.niaid.nih.gov/topics/hivaids/research/vaccines/Pages/default.aspx

General mycobacterium tuberculosis information (Lecture 19)

http://www.niaid.nih.gov/topics/tuberculosis/understanding/history/Pages/historical_killer.aspx

One Health Initiative (Lecture 11, 20)
OneHealthInitiative.com

This site explains the partnership between physicians, veterinarians, and environmentalists in their efforts to improve the health of all three. This collaboration seeks to enhance health care by combined efforts in research and treatments in all three areas.

ProMED (Lecture 24)
ProMEDmail.org

ProMED-mail is a program of the International Society for Infectious Diseases (http://www.isid.org). Get the latest updates on emerging disease outbreaks on this site.

The goal is to rapidly disseminate information on outbreaks related to human health, as well as diseases in animals and plants used for food or animal feed. They collaborate closely with HealthMap at Children's Hospital in Boston.

promed-weekly-update@promedmail.org

Skoll Foundation (Lecture 20, 24)
http://www.skollfoundation.org/news-from-the-skoll-global-threats-fund/

Larry Brilliant (M.D. and M.P.H.) and eBay's cofounder, Jeff Skoll, teamed up to put in place the Global Threats Skoll Fund, which seeks to quickly identify worldwide threats, such as Middle East peace, clean water, pandemics, climate change, and nuclear weapons. Dr. Brilliant has written many articles on pandemic threats and has worked with the World Health Organization on various projects, including the eradication of smallpox.

TED: Ideas Worth Spreading (Lecture 24)
TED.com

Known for its 18-minute (or less) talks that cover science, business, and global issues, this organization seeks to build a free knowledge clearinghouse from some of the world's experts. Its semiannual conference has been described as "the brain spa."

TED Talk: Larry Brilliant on world pandemics

https://www.ted.com/talks/larry_brilliant_wants_to_stop_pandemics/transcript

The United States President's Emergency Plan for Aids Relief (PEPFAR) (Lecture 18)
PEPFAR.gov

This site describes the goals and strategies of PEPFAR and its partners in preventing and treating AIDS.

World Health Organization (WHO) (Lecture 20)
WHO.int

This organization directs health activities for countries within the United Nations realm. This includes monitoring global health outbreaks and coordinating responses. It also provides disease outbreak updates.

Global alert response (Lecture 24)

http://www.who.int/csr/en/

WHO antibiotic crisis report 2014 (Lecture 6)

http://www.who.int/drugresistance/documents/surveillancereport/en/

Communicable disease after natural disasters (Lecture 20)

http://www.who.int/diseasecontrol_emergencies/guidelines/CD_Disasters_26_06.pdf

H5N1 influenza frequently asked questions (Lecture 21, 24)

http://www.who.int/influenza/human_animal_interface/avian_influenza/h5n1_research/faqs/en/

Peer-Reviewed Journals

The Lancet

http://www.thelancet.com/access-to-content

By registering at this site, you can access abstracts, world reports, global health content, and selected full-text articles at no cost. There is a weekly journal, as well as seven specialty journals, including *Global Health* and *Infectious Diseases*. There are also interesting blogs and podcasts available on many topics.

Emerging infectious diseases and pandemic potential: Status quo and reducing risk of global spread (Lecture 24)

http://www.thelancet.com/journals/laninf/article/PIIS1473-3099%2814%2970846-1/fulltext

Infectious diseases in Syrian conflict (Lecture 20)

http://www.thelancet.com/journals/laninf/article/PIIS1473-3099(13)70089-6/fulltext

Retraction of autism claim with vaccinations (Lecture 9)

http://www.sciencebasedmedicine.org/lancet-retracts-wakefield-article/

A wake-up call for polio eradication (Lecture 1, 3)

http://www.thelancet.com/journals/laninf/article/PIIS1473-3099%2813%2970368-2/fulltext

Public Library of Science (PLOS)

PLOS.org

A nonprofit, open-access scientific publishing project designed to create a library of open-access journals and other literature.

Reassessing Google flu trends data for detection of seasonal and pandemic influenza: A comparative epidemiological study at three geographic scales (Lecture 24)

http://www.ploscompbiol.org/article/info%3Adoi%2F10.1371%2Fjournal.pcbi.1003256

Internet Scientific Publications

ISPUB.com

An open-access collection of scientific and medical journals.

Ebola Reston: Hot zone 20 years later (Lecture 20)

http://ispub.com/IJPRM/2/1/12768

JSTOR

JSTOR.org

A digital library of academic journals and books.

Hospital attire recommendations (Lecture 17)

http://www.jstor.org/stable/10.1086/675066

Academic Organizations

Harvard Health Publications

How to boost your immune system (Lecture 10)

http://www.health.harvard.edu/flu-resource-center/how-to-boost-your-immune-system.htm

UCLA

N95 mask pros and cons (Lecture 22, 24)

http://www.ph.ucla.edu/epi/bioter/n95masks.html

Yale Environment 360

Cholera and climate change (Lecture 24)

http://e360.yale.edu/feature/climates_strong_fingerprint__in_global_cholera_outbreaks/2371/

Pandemic from wildlife (Lecture 11, 24)

http://e360.yale.edu/feature/quammen_the_next_pandemic_will_come_from_wildlife/2579/

Magazines and Newspapers

Business Insider

Human error and pandemics (Lecture 24)

http://www.businessinsider.com/our-next-pandemic-could-start-from-within-2014-7

The Guardian

The creation of pandemic viruses by U.S. labs (Lecture 24)

http://www.theguardian.com/science/2014/jun/11/crazy-dangerous-creation-deadly-airborne-flu-virus

National Geographic

Avian influenza as the next pandemic (Lecture 24)

http://ngm.nationalgeographic.com/ngm/0510/feature1/

Scientific American

Feed a cold, starve a fever (Lecture 10)

http://www.scientificamerican.com/article/fact-or-fiction-feed-a-cold/

Washington Post

Botox as bioterrorism threat (Lecture 22)

http://www.washingtonpost.com/wp-dyn/content/article/2010/01/24/AR2010012403013.html

News Shows

Global Post

Syria disease outbreaks civil war (Lecture 20)

http://www.globalpost.com/dispatch/news/regions/middle-east/syria/130221/syria-disease-outbreak-typhoid-hepatitis-A-WHO

PBS

Debunking the movie *Contagion* (Lecture 24)

http://www.pbs.org/newshour/rundown/cdc-experts-examine-the-science-of-hollywoods-contagion/

Other References

Biological weapons FAQ (Lecture 22)

http://www.fas.org/nuke/guide/usa/cbw/bw.htm

Debunking the movie *Outbreak* (Lecture 24)

http://blogs.reuters.com/great-debate/2014/08/14/remember-the-movie-outbreak-yeah-ebolas-not-really-like-that/

History of early biological warfare (Lecture 22)

http://www.chimeralinsight.com/2014/02/the-early-history-of-biological-warefare.html

Lies Hollywood taught us about Ebola and disease research (Lecture 24)

http://mic.com/articles/95372/5-big-lies-hollywood-taught-us-about-ebola-and-disease-research

General Online Sites

AIDS.gov

Timeline of HIV events (Lecture 18)

http://www.aids.gov/hiv-aids-basics/hiv-aids-101/aids-timeline/

American Academy of Physicians (AAFP.org)

Tonsil removal guidelines (Lecture 8)

http://www.aafp.org/afp/2011/0901/p566.html

The American Foundation for AIDS Research (Amfar.org)

HIV statistics (Lecture 18)

http://www.amfar.org/about-hiv-and-aids/facts-and-stats/statistics--worldwide/

Biosafety-info.net

Variola virus approval WHO research 2014 (Lecture 22)

http://www.biosafety-info.net/file_dir/129972354652e789b1524b4.pdf

European Information Networks (einiras.org)

Asia: Ground zero for the next pandemic (Lecture 24)

http://www.einiras.org/Services/Digital-Library/Publications/Detail/?lng=en&id=25174

Flu.gov

1918 pandemic influenza (Lecture 21)

http://www.flu.gov/pandemic/history/1918/the_pandemic/influenza/index.html

Pneumococcal vaccine recommendations, updated (Lecture 14)

http://www.healio.com/infectious-disease/vaccine-preventable-diseases/news/online/%7Bc6ff5151-197f-486f-86f5-11bce48197ee%7D/acip-recommends-pcv13-for-older-adults

Healthline.com

10 worst disease outbreaks in U.S. history (Lecture 23)

http://www.healthline.com/health-slideshow/10-worst-disease-outbreaks

11 dirtiest places in your home (Lecture 7)

http://www.healthline.com/health-slideshow/germy-places

Genital herpes and newspaper article history (Lecture 4, 8)

http://www.livingsphere.com/genital-herpes-and-magazines-newspapers-read-all-about-it/

U.S. Preventive Services Task Force (USpreventiveservicestaskforce.org)

Sexually transmitted disease prevention guidelines (Lecture 16)

http://www.uspreventiveservicestaskforce.org/uspstf08/methods/stinfections.htm

WEB MD (WebMD.com)

6 dirty places in your home and workplace (Lecture 7)

http://www.webmd.com/women/home-health-and-safety-9/places-germs-hide

http://www.webmd.com/news/20120523/the-6-dirtiest-work-places

Notes